THE
SOCIAL
MEDICINE
READER

Second edition

VOLUME III   Health Policy,
Markets, and
Medicine

JONATHAN OBERLANDER

LARRY R. CHURCHILL

SUE E. ESTROFF

GAIL E. HENDERSON

NANCY M. P. KING

RONALD P. STRAUSS

editors

DUKE UNIVERSITY PRESS
Durham and London 2005

© 2005 Duke University Press • All rights reserved
Printed in the United States of America on acid-free paper ∞
Typeset in Trump Mediaeval by Keystone Typesetting, Inc.
Library of Congress Cataloging-in-Publication Data
appear on the last printed page of this book.
2nd printing, 2007

Contents

Preface to the Second Edition   vii

Introduction   1

Part I   The Uninsured, Health Care Costs, and Public Programs

The U.S. Health Care System: On a Road to Nowhere?,
Jonathan Oberlander   5

Wanted: A Clearly Articulated Social Ethic for American
Health Care, *Uwe E. Reinhardt*   25

From Bismarck to Medicare—A Brief History of Medical
Care Payment in America, *Donald L. Madison*   31

The Sad History of Health Care Cost Containment as
Told in One Chart, *Drew E. Altman and Larry Levitt*   67

The Unsurprising Surprise of Renewed Health Care
Cost Inflation, *Henry J. Aaron*   70

The Not-So-Sad History of Medicare Cost Containment
as Told in One Chart, *Thomas Bodenheimer*   73

Medicaid and Medicare: The Unanticipated Politics
of Public Insurance Programs, *Lawrence D. Brown
and Michael S. Sparer*   76

Part II   Managed Care, Markets, and Rationing

Bedside Manna, *Deborah Stone*   95

Must Good HMOS Go Bad? The Commercialization of
Prepaid Group Health Care, *Robert Kuttner*   107

Defending My Life, *Geov Parrish*   119

Business vs. Medical Ethics: Conflicting Standards
for Managed Care, *Wendy K. Mariner*   128

The Prostitute, the Playboy, and the Poet: Rationing
Schemes for Organ Transplantation, *George J. Annas*   150

Ethics of Queuing for Coronary Artery Bypass Grafting
in Canada, *Jafna L. Cox*   158

Rationing in Practice: The Case of In Vitro Fertilization,
Sharon Redmayne and Rudolf Klein   167

Part III   International Perspectives and Emerging Issues

Reforming the Health Care System: The Universal
Dilemma, *Uwe E. Reinhardt*   179

Health Care in Four Nations, *Thomas Bodenheimer
and Kevin Grumbach*   199

Keeping Quality on the Policy Agenda,
Elizabeth A. McGlynn and Robert H. Brook   230

What's Ahead for Health Insurance in the United States?,
Victor R. Fuchs   240

Luxury Primary Care—Market Innovation or Threat
to Access?, *Troyen A. Brennan*   246

Correspondence: Response to "Luxury Primary Care"   255

Limiting Health Care for the Old, *Daniel Callahan*   260

Scapegoating the Aged: Intergenerational Equity and
Age-Based Rationing, *Robert H. Binstock*   267

Index to Authors   285

About the Editors   287

Preface to the Second Edition

Of the six editors of this second edition of the *Social Medicine Reader*, five are current members and one a former member of the Department of Social Medicine, University of North Carolina at Chapel Hill School of Medicine. Founded in 1977, the Department of Social Medicine includes scholars in medicine, the social sciences, the humanities, and public health. Its mission is to inform the work and thought of researchers, teachers, and practitioners on the social conditions and characteristics of patients, causes of illness, and barriers to effective care; and the responsibilities of the medical profession and other medical institutions.

This reader is based on the syllabus of a year-long, required, interdisciplinary course, Medicine and Society, which has been taught to first-year students at the University of North Carolina at Chapel Hill School of Medicine since 1978. The goal of the course since its inception has been to demonstrate that medicine and medical practice have a profound influence on—and are influenced by—social, cultural, political, and economic forces. Teaching this perspective requires integrating medical and nonmedical materials and viewpoints. This reader, therefore, arises not from one or two academic disciplines, but from many fields within medicine, the social sciences, and humanities.

With health care and health so central to the political, personal, and financial discourse of the day, this reader provides a starting point for informed, critical analysis. The three volumes of the *Social Medicine Reader* represent the most engaging, provocative, and informative materials and issues we have traversed with our students. While the origin of these volumes lies in the teaching of medical students, the selections were deliberately made with an eye toward engaging nonmedical readers, both from the interested public and from students in the arts and sciences.

The selections challenge standard ways of thinking about medical categories of disease, social categories of risk, and the types of moral reasoning on which much of the field of bioethics has been based. Their many voices include individual narratives of illness experience, commentaries by physicians, debate about complex medical cases, and conceptually and empirically based writings by scholars in medicine, the social sciences, and humanities. These are readings with the literary and scholarly power to convey the complicated relationships between medicine, health, and society. They do not resolve the most vexing contemporary issues, but illuminate them.

Medicine's impact on society is multidimensional. Biomedical technology and practice, including its latest expression, genomic medicine, have profoundly affected our institutions and our social relations. Medicine has affected how we think about the most fundamental, enduring human experiences—conception, birth, maturation, sickness, suffering, healing, aging, and death—and it has shaped the metaphors we use to express our deepest concerns. Medical practices and our responses to them have helped to redefine the meaning of age, race, and gender. Technological advances in medicine have produced ethical dilemmas expressed in new vocabularies of science and economics, as well as in the familiar languages of morality and human relationships.

Social influences on medicine are apparent in several ways. First, modern science presumes that the pursuit of knowledge can and should be conducted with an unwavering adherence to neutral, objective observation and experimentation. Yet medical knowledge and practice, like all knowledge and practice, is shaped by political, cultural, and economic forces, within which doctors' ideas about disease—in fact their very definitions of disease—depend on the roles science and scientists play in particular cultures, as well as on the cultures of laboratory and clinical science. Medicine tends to reduce the world to a vocabulary of its own, one that seems immune to the vagaries and vicissitudes of culture. But diseases are not immutable; they are shaped by person, time, and place, and are identified and endowed with significance only within social and cultural contexts.

Despite the power of the biomedical model of disease and the increasing specificity of molecular and genetic knowledge, social factors have always influenced the occurrence and course of most diseases. And once disease has occurred, the power of medicine to alter its course is constrained by the larger social and economic context. Beyond these problems, many medical interventions are themselves of contested or unclear value. Spending on health care in the United States has long outstripped that of other industrialized nations, but that spending has not resulted in a healthier population. What does our medicine produce? Who benefits from these enormous expenditures of resources?

Repeatedly, the readings throughout these three volumes make clear that much of what we encounter in science, in society, and in everyday and extraordinary lives is indeterminate, ambiguous, complex, and contradictory. And because of this inherent ambiguity, the interwoven selections highlight conflicts—conflict about power and authority, autonomy and choice, security and risk. By critically analyzing these and many other related issues, we can open up possibilities, change what seems inevitable, and practice medical education and doctoring with an increased capacity for reflection and self-examination. The goal is to ignite and to fuel the inner voices of social, human, and moral analysis among health care professionals, and among us all.

Any collection of readings like the three volumes that make up the *Social Medicine Reader* is open to challenges about what has been included and what has been left out. This collection is no exception. The study of medicine and society is dynamic, with large and ever expanding bodies of new literature from which to draw. We have omitted some readings widely considered "classics" and included some readings that are classic only in our experience. We have chosen to include material with literary and scholarly merit and that has worked well in the classroom, provoking discussion and engaging readers' imaginations. These readings invite self-conscious, multilevel, critical examination, a work of reading and discussion that is inherently difficult but educationally rewarding.

The first edition of the *Social Medicine Reader* was a single volume. We decided to make the second edition three volumes to facilitate use by different audiences with different interests; however, the three volumes also function as an integrated whole. Volume I, *Patients, Doctors, and Illness*, examines the experience of illness, the roles and training of health care professionals and their relationships with patients, ethics in health care, and experiences and decisions at the end of life. It includes fictional and nonfiction narratives and poetry; definitions and case-based discussions of moral precepts in health care, such as truth telling, informed consent, privacy, autonomy, and beneficence; and scholarly readings providing legal, ethical, and practical perspectives on many familiar but persistent ethical and social questions raised by illness and health care. Volume II, *Social and Cultural Contributions to Health, Difference, and Inequality*, explores health and illness, focusing on how difference and disability are defined and experienced in contemporary America and how the social categories commonly used to predict disease outcomes—gender, race/ ethnicity, and social class—have become contested terrain. Narratives and essays feature individuals managing illness in daily life, and families both coping with and contributing to the challenges of ill health. Social epidemiological categories are examined empirically and critically. Volume III, *Health Policy, Markets, and Medicine,* examines issues and controversies in health policy. Essays analyze a broad spectrum of topics, from the historical forces that shaped development of the American health system to contemporary reform debates over controlling medical care spending and covering the uninsured. International health systems, medical care rationing, and emerging policy issues—including the rise of consumer-driven insurance and population aging—are also explored.

We thank our teaching colleagues who helped create and refine both the first and the second editions of this reader. These colleagues have come over the years from both within and outside the Department of Social Medicine and the University of North Carolina at Chapel Hill. Equal gratitude goes to our students, whose criticism and enthusiasm over two decades have improved our teaching and have influenced us greatly in making the selections for the Reader. The leadership of Department of Social Medicine chairs and course directors since 1978 has also been invaluable. We thank the department's faculty and staff, past and present; we especially thank Judy Benoit, for many years the Medicine and Society course coordinator, and Jeff Kim, our student research assistant. In addition, Larry Churchill thanks the faculty who have taught with him in the Ecology of Health Care course at Vanderbilt School of Medicine during 2002 and 2003 for their many ideas for improving the second edition of the reader. Jon Oberlander gratefully acknowledges the support of the Greenwall Foundation and its Faculty Scholars Program in Bioethics. The editors gratefully acknowledge support from the Department of Social Medicine, University of North Carolina at Chapel Hill School of Medicine, and the Center for Clinical and Research Ethics, Vanderbilt University.

Health Policy, Markets, and Medicine

Introduction

Health care has become a perennial issue in American politics. Since 1970, the American health care system has grappled with an unsettling combination of rapidly rising costs and a growing uninsured population, prompting both multiple declarations of crisis and efforts at reform. This has been a turbulent period in health policy: the past four decades have seen dramatic changes in private health insurance, campaigns to enact national health insurance, and the rise (and perhaps fall) of managed care. Yet public and private initiatives have so far failed either to stem medical care inflation or to guarantee universal coverage. The American health system is in constant motion, but for all its innovation, solutions have proved elusive.

This book volume III of the *Social Medicine Reader* series—explores major issues and controversies in health policy. Our approach is interdisciplinary: the selections in this volume reflect a wide range of perspectives, including those of political science, economics, history, bioethics, medicine, and health services research. This diversity illuminates the many ways that scholars think about health policy and invites readers to investigate a broad spectrum of issues, from the origins of private insurance to the future of health reform. *Health Policy, Markets, and Medicine* is intended for a wide audience. We have chosen readings that are accessible, insightful, and provocative. These selections have been taught successfully in a number of health policy courses, and this volume is designed for use in undergraduate, medical school, public health, and public policy classes.

Readings in part I address issues of the uninsured, health care costs, and public insurance programs. We begin with essays that review the history of American health policy, explain the contours of the current system and the ethical implications of our insurance system, and assess recent incremental efforts at reform. These selections introduce themes in the politics of health care and uncover the historical as well as moral foundations of today's health policy debates. Subsequent readings in this section examine why health care spending has proven so hard to control in the United States, and elaborate the political dynamics of Medicare and Medicaid.

Part II focuses on managed care, markets, and rationing. Because the United States has a system that relies on private insurance, changes in health policy are often driven by the private sector. In recent years, market-led reform has transformed health insurance and medical practice. Essays in this section explore the rise of managed care, its impact on patients and physicians, and the ethical implications of applying a business ethos to medical care. This section also highlights controversies in health care rationing, an issue that, as the readings make clear, is central to all modern health systems. The authors explore how scarce resources can be allocated fairly and the ethics of imposing limits on medical care services.

Part III continues the comparative theme by providing an international perspective on health reform, with essays that compare the American approach to health policy and its underlying philosophical foundations with European countries, Canada, and Japan. Additional readings probe emerging policy issues, including the post–managed care wave of consumer-driven health care, and efforts to move quality of care to the top of the agenda. The American health care system is, of course, a moving target with an uncertain future; this makes predictions about what's next a risky endeavor. This caveat notwithstanding, the section concludes with a set of readings that debate the one issue that is almost certain to resonate in coming decades: the implications for public policy of the aging of America and whether the United States can afford the medical care bill for the baby-boom generation.

PART I

**The Uninsured, Health Care Costs,
and Public Programs**

The U.S. Health Care System: On a Road to Nowhere?

Jonathan Oberlander

The health care system in the United States remains a "paradox of excess and deprivation."[1] The United States spends more on medical services than any other nation, and U.S. physicians earn more than their counterparts in Canada, Europe, and Japan. An extraordinary amount of money—as much as $300 billion annually—goes to pay just for the system's administrative costs.[2] Americans with insurance have access to the latest in sophisticated medical technology and innovative medical procedures; rates of diffusion for many medical technologies, such as magnetic resonance imaging, are higher in the United States than in other countries.[3] Indeed, the availability of these resources is so widespread that some analysts believe that well-insured Americans receive too many medical services.

At the same time, millions of Americans receive too little medical care.[4] Over 40 million (and counting) Americans do not have health insurance, which makes the United States the only industrial democracy in the world with a substantial uninsured population. Even those with health insurance may be underinsured, lacking both coverage for key services and adequate financial protection against the costs of medical care.

The 1990s was a decade of great expectations in U.S. health policy—expectations that ultimately were not met. Health reform efforts in both the public and private sectors failed to resolve the major problems in American medical care. In 1993, President Bill Clinton proposed a government-sponsored system of universal health insurance, but despite initial optimism about its political prospects, the bill failed in Congress. After

Jonathan Oberlander, "The U.S. Health Care System: On a Road to Nowhere?," from *Canadian Medical Association Journal*, vol. 167, 163–168. © 2002 by the Canadian Medical Association. Reprinted by permission of the publisher.

the defeat of the Clinton plan, the private market emerged as the engine of health care reform. The U.S. health insurance system moved toward "managed care" arrangements, with rising enrollment in health maintenance organizations (HMOs) and the growth of for-profit health plans. Proponents touted market-based reform as a solution to health care cost inflation and an opportunity to enhance both quality of care and patient choice. However, by decade's end a widespread backlash against managed care had developed, initial success in controlling costs had abated, and managed care's appeal as the latest magic bullet in American health policy was waning.

What is the state of the U.S. health care system after a decade of turbulence? What political dynamics are driving health policy? And what is the outlook for health care reform? This essay introduces readers to issues in American health policy, and reviews the contemporary politics and future prospects of health care reform. In particular I focus on the persistent problem of the uninsured, efforts at cost control and incremental reform, and the rise and fall of managed care.

Little Progress for the Uninsured

The U.S. health care system is often erroneously labeled a private health care system. In fact, the United States has a mixed system of public and private insurance, though the word "system" connotes much more organization, rationale, and logic than is actually at work. Most working-age Americans receive health insurance through their employers (table 1).[5] This private insurance is voluntary in the sense that companies are not required by law to provide health coverage, though employer-based insurance is subsidized by federal tax policies (employers' premium contributions are tax exempt) at an annual cost to the government of over $100 billion in foregone revenues.[6] Medicare, a federal government program, provides health insurance to virtually all Americans over 65 years of age, as well as to persons with disabilities and end-stage renal disease. Medicaid, a jointly funded federal-state program, pays for medical services for low-income Americans (though it covers only about 40% of the poor), including seniors who spend down their incomes and assets to a level that qualifies them for Medicaid-funded nursing home care. In between those covered by this hodgepodge of private and public plans, however, lies a substantial population without any health insurance at all.

In 2003, 45 million Americans—15.6% of the population—lacked health

Table 1. Sources of Health Insurance Coverage in the United States, 2002

Type of Coverage	Population Covered, % *
Any private plan	69.6
Employer-based plan	61.3
Government plan	25.7
Medicare	13.4
Medicaid	11.6
Military plan	3.5
None	15.2

Source: Source of data is US Census Bureau
* Total is not 100%, because some people have multiple sources of insurance.

insurance.[7] About 80% of the uninsured are workers or live in families with workers. They typically have low-wage jobs or work in small businesses in which the employer does not offer health insurance or, if it is offered, they cannot afford to purchase it.[8] However, a growing share of the uninsured population is employed by large firms, a trend explained primarily by the decline in manufacturing jobs and reduced rates of unionization;[9] companies such as Wal-Mart, the largest private employer in the United States, employ eligibility restrictions and long waiting periods on insurance coverage for part-time workers.[10] The uninsured are also disproportionately of low income. In 2002, one-third of the poor were uninsured and nearly two-thirds of the uninsured had incomes less than 200% of the federal poverty line, or $29,000 for a family of 3.[11] A substantially higher percentage of black (20%) and Hispanic (32%) than white (14%) Americans were uninsured in 2002.[12]

Many Americans mistakenly believe that the uninsured obtain adequate medical care from hospital emergency rooms and other charity sources. Studies have consistently found, however, that the uninsured receive much less medical care than insured Americans.[13] Nearly 25% of uninsured children and 40% of uninsured adults have no regular source of medical care.[14] The uninsured are much more likely to delay or forego needed treatment, have their conditions diagnosed at a later stage, and be admitted to hospitals for avoidable conditions; overall, the uninsured use 50% fewer medical services than those with private insurance.[15] The Institute of Medicine estimates that 18,000 uninsured Americans die each year prematurely due to a lack of access to proper medical care.[16] Moreover, inadequate insurance coverage carries with it financial as well as

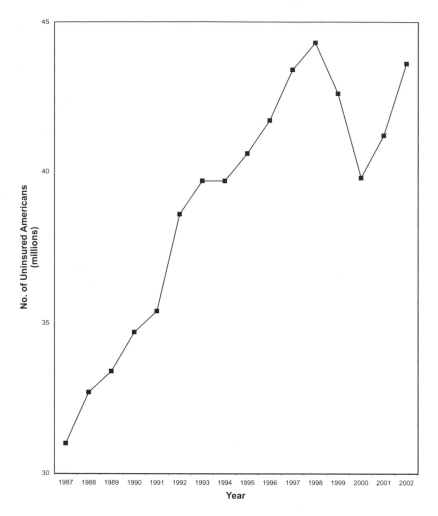

Figure 1. Number of Uninsured Americans, 1987–2002.

medical risks: the costs of medical treatment are a leading cause of bank-ruptcy in the United States.[17] Indeed, about half of all bankruptcies in the United States "involve a medical reason or large medical debt."[18]

The number of uninsured Americans has climbed steadily upward since the 1980s (figure 1). During 1998–1999, though, the uninsured population declined from 44.3 million to 42.6 million, and in 2000, fell again to 39.8 million (though this drop was due in part to statistical adjustments in how the government counted the uninsured). Yet perhaps most striking was not the decrease, but rather that it took so long to happen and that the overall trend during the decade remained one of an expanding uninsured population. During much of the 1990s the United States enjoyed ideal conditions for an expansion of health insurance. The economy went through an unprecedented era of sustained growth, the rates of general inflation and unemployment were both exceptionally low, and health care inflation moderated. Still, from 1990 to 1999 the number of uninsured Americans increased by nearly 8 million.

That even these favorable circumstances did not generate any significant expansion of health insurance was disquieting. It also revealed the limits of the market and the voluntary health insurance system, left to their own devices, to solve or even substantially ameliorate the problem of the uninsured. Nor did it bode well for the future when the inevitable economic downturn would come and pressure the employment-based health insurance system. Indeed, economic growth slowed in 2000, and in 2001 in the aftermath of the September 11 attacks, the United States entered a recession with substantially higher rates of unemployment. The predictable result of job loss was a sharp increase in the ranks of the uninsured: in 2002, the number of uninsured Americans rose by 2.4 million, the biggest one-year increase in America's uninsured population since 1992.[19]

In coming years, a reenergized economy could well slow the rate of growth in the uninsured population, but it will not reverse the long-term trend. For the foreseeable future, the number of uninsured Americans is likely to continue to grow absent government action.

The Politics of Health Insurance

National health insurance periodically emerged on the U.S. political agenda during the 20th century and occasionally was tantalizingly close to enactment. The most recent failure came in 1994, with the defeat of the Health Security Act, sponsored by President Bill Clinton (and drafted under the guidance of his wife, Hillary Rodham Clinton). President Clinton proposed to achieve universal coverage in the United States by mandating that all employers provide private health insurance to their employees and by giving small businesses and unemployed Americans subsidies with which to purchase insurance. However, the Clinton plan triggered fierce opposition from the insurance industry (which disliked the proposed limits on their profits and regulation of behaviors, such as experience rating, that enabled them to charge higher premiums for sick patients), the business community (which criticized the employer mandate), ideological conservatives (who saw the plan as an unwarranted nationalization of the health care system), and large segments of the public (who were anxious about the plan's emphasis on moving patients into HMOs). Confronted with this opposition, and despite Democratic Party majorities in both the House of Representatives and Senate, the Clinton health plan—along with all other compromise proposals—was defeated. The American Medical Association, which initially endorsed and then waffled on the idea of universal coverage, did not play a prominent role in the 1993–1994 debate, a sign of its deteriorating influence on U.S. health politics.

One legacy of the Clinton plan's failure was caution regarding health policy. Most politicians took the lesson of the plan's demise to be that comprehensive reform was not politically feasible. Consequently, from 1994 to 2003 talk of attaining universal coverage all but disappeared from the political landscape. Neither of the two major parties' presidential candidates in the 2000 election, Al Gore and George W. Bush, offered plans that would cover all or even most of the uninsured. Nor did any legislation for universal coverage that had a serious chance of passing emanate from Congress during this decade. One of the only organized advocacy groups for the uninsured, Families USA, even toned down its calls for universal coverage in favor of more modest policy goals.

What was remarkable about the absence of proposals for universal coverage during the period 1999–2001 was that fiscal circumstances appeared conducive to their adoption. After two decades of budget deficits, the federal government in 2000 ran a sizeable budget surplus, projected at $5.6 trillion over the next decade.[20] It had long been assumed that the lack of affordability of a public program was a central barrier to universal coverage, particularly during an era of sizeable federal deficits in which large spending increases for domestic programs were politically constrained and tax increases considered taboo. Now, though, the affordability argument was exposed as a fallacy. Despite the availability of a budget surplus that could have been used to pay the costs of covering the uninsured, universal coverage did not surface as a central political issue in 2000. Instead, political attention focused on proposals for improving the medical experiences of the already insured through regulation of managed care and expansion of Medicare to cover outpatient prescription drugs.

It is clear, then, that the most relevant fact about U.S. health politics is not that 15% of the population is uninsured but that 85% of Americans are insured. Those who are insured are generally satisfied with their own medical care, even if they think poorly of the system as a whole; consequently, they are not a reliable constituency for change. Indeed, any reform that threatens to alter the medical care arrangements of the well insured is likely to provoke public opposition. The formidable con- stituency—led by the insurance industry—against reform is mobilized, wealthy, and politically influential. Meanwhile, the uninsured are dispro- portionately low-income, unorganized, and apparently politically expend- able. As the Clinton plan vividly demonstrated, the political benefits to a president and legislators willing to take on a $2 trillion health care indus- try that literally profits from the status quo and opposes reform are uncer- tain, but the political costs are certain to be high. The result is that uni- versal coverage remains an elusive reform in the United States, and the uninsured continue to live in an "aura of invisibility."[21]

Incremental Reforms

In the aftermath of the Clinton plan's defeat, there was little appetite for comprehensive reforms that would assure universal coverage. One consequence was resort to a familiar foundation of American political life: federalism. By virtue of federal inaction, states became the locus for health care reform, as Oregon, Vermont, and Tennessee, among others, implemented ambitious reforms to expand access to health insurance.[22] Focused largely on extending coverage to low-income children and adults, these reforms represented a political success story when contrasted with the deadlock over health policy in Washington, D.C. However, while some states achieved noteworthy reductions in their uninsured rate, no state came close to attaining universal coverage; initial aspirations for coverage gains and cost savings were often not met, and economic trou- bles and budgetary shortfalls created pressures that threatened the sus- tainability of much-heralded state programs like the Oregon Health Plan and Tenncare. In 2002, none of the aforementioned reform-minded states had uninsured rates lower than 9%.[23] There appeared to be very real lim- its, then, to the potential of state-led health reform to cope with the uninsured problem.

At the federal level, incrementalism was in vogue. In 1996 Congress adopted the Health Insurance Portability and Accountability Act (HIPAA), which was designed to limit preexisting condition exclusion periods and make it easier for workers losing group coverage to purchase health insurance on the individual market. However, the law's insurance market reforms did not address the affordability of individual market health policies, limiting its impact on the uninsured. In 1997, Congress enacted the State Children's Health Insurance Program (SCHIP), which targeted children who lived in families with incomes below 200% of the federal poverty line but who were not eligible for Medicaid. By 2003, 4 million children were enrolled in SCHIP (funded through a federal block grant to the states), and the program helped reduce the percentage of uninsured low-income children by one-third between 1997 and 2002.[24] However, faced with severe budget shortfalls, following the 2001 recession some states instituted enrollment freezes and waiting lists for children applying for SCHIP, potentially "undermin[ing] further progress toward reducing this number."[25]

Since the enactment of SCHIP and HIPAA two main pathways to incremental health reform have emerged. The first approach, generally favored by Democrats, is to expand existing public insurance programs, including Medicaid and SCHIP. Proponents of this approach would change eligibility requirements for these programs, opening them up to more of the poor and near-poor (e.g., to parents of children enrolled in SCHIP). One of the more ambitious plans would extend Medicaid and SCHIP coverage, without premiums or cost-sharing, to all persons with incomes below 150% of the federal poverty line and subsidize enrollment for persons up to 300%.[26] It is estimated that this plan would extend eligibility for public insurance to over 25 million Americans who are currently uninsured.

Most plans, however, would not expand eligibility so broadly and would thus not reach most of the uninsured. Reforms that expand existing public programs confront another serious problem: their coverage gains may look better on paper than the subsequent reality. Millions of eligible persons for Medicaid and SCHIP are not enrolled in the programs, due to a combination of confusing eligibility standards, complex applications and enrollment processes, and underfunded outreach efforts. In 2000, for example, an estimated 84% of the 6.7 million uninsured low-income children in the United States were eligible for Medicaid or SCHIP but not enrolled in the programs.[27] Without some sort of automatic or default enrollment provision, there is every chance that the actual increase in coverage promised by incremental reforms that expand eligibility for existing public programs will fall short of the projected gains.

A second approach to incremental reform—one generally preferred by

Republicans—is to adopt tax credits that would help the uninsured purchase private insurance. This approach appears to be especially attractive given the political appeal of tax cuts and the promise of expanded coverage with minimal government involvement. Most tax cut proposals would target individuals, though some plans have instead focused on credits for employers. Tax credits could be made refundable, so that even low-income persons who do not pay federal income taxes would be eligible.

However, there are also problems with tax-credit proposals. The main problem is the mismatch between the size of the proposed tax credits and the cost of health insurance. In 2003, the average annual premium of an employer-sponsored health insurance plan in the United States cost $9,068 for family and $3,383 for individual coverage.[28] President Bush's 2004 tax credit plan proposed a maximum tax credit of up to $1,000 for individuals and $3,000 for families toward the purchase of non–group health insurance. It is questionable how much difference these tax credits would make to the uninsured, many of whom have little disposable income. This is especially true because insurance on the individual insurance market has much higher administrative costs than employer-sponsored group insurance, and consequently higher premiums (as well as generally more limited benefits). Without much higher subsidies, tax credits are not likely to reach most of the uninsured.

More fundamentally, neither tax credits nor expanded public insurance does anything to control the costs of medical care. Politically, the absence of cost control in incremental reforms is not surprising. After all, health care costs equal the total incomes of the providers of medical care, a group comprising not merely physicians but also insurers, hospitals, nursing homes, pharmaceutical companies, and all those selling medical services and products. Any attempt to restrain national health spending is viewed by providers as an assault on their livelihood, triggering intense opposition. A plausible reading of the Clinton reform debacle is that while expanding coverage is difficult, simultaneously mandating spending controls is political suicide.[29]

Yet the era of moderate medical care inflation that made inattention to cost control comfortable in the mid-1990s has ended. Absent cost control, incremental reforms may become self-defeating: higher rates of medical care inflation could lead to growing numbers of uninsured persons and higher than expected program costs, making expansion of insurance coverage less affordable, more politically problematic, and ultimately undercutting prior incremental gains in coverage. Higher costs for medical care would also increase the gap between the size of tax credits and the price of health insurance.

The Rise of Managed Care

U.S. medical care has long been the most expensive in the world, thanks to higher prices and provider incomes, greater administrative costs, and more extensive use of some costly medical procedures and technologies than other nations.[30,31] The defeat of comprehensive health reform in 1994 did not obviate the pressures to control health spending; rather, it shifted the engine of control to the private sector. Employers looking to hold down their medical bills embraced managed care and, in a staggeringly short time, managed care became the norm in U.S. health insurance. By 2000, 92% of persons with employer-sponsored insurance were enrolled in a managed care plan.[32] Managed care also spread to public programs for the poor, elderly, and disabled—Medicare and Medicaid—though enrollment of elderly Medicare beneficiaries in such plans was far lower than for the employer-sponsored population.[33]

"Managed care" came to refer to a wide range of health plans and practices that departed from the traditional American model of insurance. In the traditional model, insured patients chose their physician; physicians treated patients with absolute clinical autonomy; insurers generally paid physicians whatever they billed on a fee-for-service basis; and employers paid premiums for their workers to private insurers, footing the bill regardless of the cost. Managed care altered all of these arrangements. As a consequence of not having national health insurance, cost control in the United States focused more on setting limits on the individual medical encounter ("managing care") than on establishing budgetary limits for the entire health care sector.

The rise of managed care brought about four major changes in U.S. medical care. First was the substantial decline in traditional insurance arrangements, which allowed unfettered access to physicians and unregulated delivery of medical care. The proportion of Americans with employer-sponsored indemnity coverage declined from 95% in 1978 to 14% by 1998.[34] This drop was accompanied by an increase in enrollment in a wide variety of managed-care insurance programs, including HMOs, preferred provider organizations (PPOs), and point of service plans (POS). Not only did HMOs grow in enrollment—from 36.5 million in 1990 to 58.2

million in 1995—but they also changed substantially in form. In particular, there was rapid growth in for-profit HMOS as well as network and individual-practice association (IPA) models that contracted with providers; in contrast group or staff-model HMOS (such as Kaiser Permanente) owned their facilities, and physicians worked exclusively for them.[35] Yet, while they continued to be regarded as the symbol of managed care, the growth of HMOS stalled in the late 1990s, and by 2003, PPOS covered more than twice as many Americans (54%) with employer-provided insurance than HMOS (24%).[36]

Second, patients in managed care received full coverage for services only if they chose a physician within the plan's network. In the case of HMOS, patients generally received no coverage if they saw an out-of-network provider. In some plans, patients had to go through a gatekeeper, typically a primary care physician, to obtain a specialty referral. The corollary was that many insurers no longer contracted with all physicians in a community. Rather, they selectively contracted with a limited number of doctors, negotiating price discounts in exchange for guaranteed patient volume and excluding high-cost providers.

Third, physicians' decisions were regularly subject to external review by insurance plans. Indeed, U.S. physicians probably experienced more intrusion into their clinical lives than physicians anywhere in the industrialized world, an ironic development given that the American Medical Association long opposed national health insurance as a threat to clinical autonomy.[37] Under utilization review arrangements, physicians had to seek permission from the patient's insurance company for admission to a hospital, diagnostic tests, or medical procedures. Utilization review and physician profiling also occurred after treatment, with the goal of identifying "inappropriate" or "excessive" care according to the insurer's standards. Proponents of managed care argued that these practices could not only control costs but also enhance quality of care—for instance, by assuring adherence to evidence-based medicine and eliminating medically unnecessary services.

Fourth, insurers no longer gave physicians a blank check; instead, they dictated not only what doctors were paid but also how they were paid. This led to the widespread adoption of predetermined fee schedules for physician payment by managed care plans, which sought discounts from "normal" fees. HMOS also adopted capitated payment, often focusing on primary care providers. Under capitated payment, physicians received a set amount for each patient enrolled in their practice, regardless of that patient's actual use of services. The stated aim was to avoid the financial incentive for overtreatment inherent in fee-for-service payment. Another important change in payment arrangements was the introduction of bonuses and other incentives for physicians to meet targets in providing care. Frequently these incentives were aimed at ensuring that physicians held down costs in a capitated environment; for instance, bonuses were provided to physicians whose rate of admission to hospital for their patient pool was lower than the insurer's target. Along with capitation, these arrangements put the incomes of many physicians at substantial risk.[38]

The Impact of Managed Care on Costs and Quality

After the spread of managed care in the early 1990s, health care spending in the United States slowed (table 2). From 1993 to 1998, the share of gross domestic product (GDP) devoted to national health spending declined from 13.7% to 13.5%, and premiums for employer-sponsored health insurance actually grew more slowly than per capita GDP.[39] From 1994 to 1997, per capita medical care spending rose by an annual average of 2.4%. In historical terms, this was a period of remarkable restraint in U.S. medical spending, though the United States continued to spend far more on medical care than any other nation.[40,41]

There was substantial disagreement among analysts about the significance of the relative success of the United States in controlling health care spending during the mid-1990s. Some observers believed that this experience demonstrated managed care's effectiveness in controlling costs and the efficiencies inherent in strategies such as selective contracting, utilization review and capitation. Others attributed the slowdown to a one-time switch from indemnity insurance that could not be duplicated or to temporary circumstances that could not be sustained, such as marketing strategies that led insurers to underprice their products to expand market share. The long-term cost-containment potential of managed care consequently remained uncertain. Beginning in 1999 health care spending once again rose at higher rates and during the period 1999–2002, per capita spending on medical services increased by an annual average rate of 8.6%, more than three times the rate of general inflation.[42] The end of the short-lived era of low medical care inflation suggested that managed care's ability to restrain spending had been exaggerated.

Evidence for the impact of managed care on the quality of care during the 1990s was mixed. Most studies found little difference in quality

Table 2. Changes in Annual per Capita Spending on Medical Care
and Employer-based Health Insurance Premiums, 1991–2003

| | Annual Change, % | |
Year	Medical Care Spending	Employer-based Insurance Premiums*
1991	6.9%	11.5%
1992	6.6	10.9
1993	5.0	8.5
1994	2.1	4.8
1995	2.2	2.3
1996	2.0	0.8
1997	3.3	2.1
1998	5.3	3.7
1999	7.1	4.8
2000	7.8	8.3
2001	10.0	11.0
2002	9.5	12.7
2003	7.4	13.9

Source: Source of data is Center for Studying Health System Change.
*For 1991–1992, 1994, and 1997, premium data are based on large firms only; for all other years the data are for all firms.

of care between traditional insurers and managed care plans, though there was some evidence of worse outcomes for chronically ill seniors in HMOs.[43] In addition, higher rates of managed care plans' market penetration were associated with physicians providing lower rates of charity and uncompensated care to uninsured patients.[44]

That quality of medical care in many cases did not deteriorate, despite reduced volume and intensity of services, suggested that the previous standard of "unmanaged" care incorporated significant amounts of unnecessary services. However, these findings also cast doubt on the premise that managed care was improving quality through practice guidelines, preventive care, primary care, disease management, integrated delivery systems, and other strategies. Too often, these strategies existed more as marketing labels than as workable or proven innovations, though that did not stop them from being aggressively promoted outside the United States, often to receptive audiences overseas looking for new levers to control costs and improve quality and consumer service. Yet managed care plans in the United States had not consistently implemented these practices, and market competition did not result in significant quality

improvements. Instead, plans focused on managing costs, a decision reinforced by employers, who were much more likely to select insurance on
the basis of price than on the basis of quality.[45]

The End of Managed Care?

Regardless of the evidence, there was strong sentiment among both physicians and patients that managed care was harming quality of care. Consequently, a backlash against managed care emerged, culminating in a push
to enact patients' bills of rights and other laws that regulated the behavior
of managed care plans.[46] In the 1990s, the 50 U.S. states adopted 900 such
laws, including reforms that established procedures for appealing health
plan decisions, assured coverage of emergency room visits, banned "gag
clauses" that prevented physicians from discussing treatment options,
and guaranteed access to specialists.[47] These laws were popular with legislators precisely because they served to reassure the voting public that
something was being done about HMO abuses, though the effectiveness of
many of these provisions was uncertain. The issue also drew national
political attention in the late 1990s, but Congress deadlocked over competing versions of a Patient's Bill of Rights and failed to pass a bill.

Legislative activity, however, was not the only source or sign of growing
disenchantment with managed care. By the end of the 1990s, managed
care plans, in reaction to patient and doctor complaints, were loosening
many of their restrictions on health care utilization, such as gatekeeping
requirements, and broadening previously restricted physician and hospital networks.[48] The decline in HMO enrollment and shift to looser insurance arrangements like PPOs was another indication of dissatisfaction
with managed care's constraints on access to medical care. PPOs were
commonly regarded by analysts as an insurance model "particularly inca-
pable of managing quality or cost,"[49] and arguably had more in common
with traditional insurance than they did with HMOs. Employers, who had
triggered the managed care revolution, also retreated from their embrace
of HMOs and aim of managing workers' medical experiences, partly in response to tight labor market conditions that advantaged workers.[50] Thus
the vision of managed care ushering in a new world in American medical
care, a system of integrated health plans based on capitation, managed
competition, and quality innovation had been, at best, deferred; others
saw it as having collapsed altogether.[51]

The cause of managed care's deteriorating ability to hold down costs was again debated, with some analysts blaming the politically inspired managed care backlash or providers' success in consolidating to gain market power and economic leverage over health plans. Others argued managed care's ability to slow health spending always had been exaggerated and that it did little to stem the most important long-term factor in rising costs: development and diffusion of costly medical technology. Nor did managed care do much, critics argued, to curtail the prohibitive administrative costs of American medicine. In any case, as managed care lost its capacity to control costs, the willingness of key constituencies to tolerate its limitations, which has been tenuous even at its apex, evaporated.

By 2001 managed care's future appeared sufficiently bleak that one prominent analyst declared the "end of managed care."[52] This may well be a premature declaration—despite the backlash, the U.S. health care system has not gone back to what it was before. HMOS continue to be a significant presence in U.S. health insurance and many managed care practices remain prevalent. Indeed, interest in some forms of care management still appears to be growing. There is ongoing development, for instance, of quality initiatives that manage the care of chronically ill patients. And rising levels of medical care spending and insurance premiums could lead to a resurgence of managed care-style cost controls, perhaps under a politically more palatable label such as "enhanced care." To be sure, though, the confidence that managed care can swiftly cure the ills of American medicine which characterized the early 1990s has been lost.

Conclusion

After a decade of much anticipated changes and largely failed efforts at health reform, the United States appears to be no closer to solving the problems of cost control and access that have characterized its health care system for the past three decades. The number of uninsured is once again marching ever upward, and after the experiment with managed care and market competition, health care spending is again climbing at a steep rate.[53] Where does health reform in the United States go from here?

The market is already moving past managed care onto the next supposed magic bullet: consumer-driven health care. Under this rubric a variety of trends are touted, including the proliferation of Web-based medical information and Internet technology that allows employees to tailor their own custom-made health benefits packages and provider networks.[54]

Consumer-driven health care also refers to health insurance arrangements that combine high-deductible catastrophic coverage with medical or health savings accounts to pay for "routine" expenditures. While such arrangements have potential appeal for healthy and wealthy patients (as well as employers looking to limit their annual health care bill to a defined contribution), they will not help high-cost, chronically ill patients who desire more health security and could be hit hard financially by higher deductibles. As a result, if consumer-driven plans spread in employer-provided insurance, the American health insurance system could further segment on the basis of health risk.[55]

Another market trend (often grouped under the same banner of consumerism) is rising patient cost-sharing in the form of increases in employees' share of premiums, as well as higher deductibles and larger copayments that may vary according to patients' choice of hospitals or physicians from tiered (differentially priced) networks of medical care providers.[56] The focus on increasing cost sharing (known as "buying down" coverage) represents a tool for employers looking to limit their bill for rising insurance premiums, as well as a shift away from HMOs' earlier efforts to limit financial barriers to primary care. While increasing patient cost-sharing may not constrain overall inflation in medical care, it nonetheless appeals to companies as an effective form of cost shifting that moves the burden of rising health costs onto employees.[57]

Consumer-driven health care is thus the magic bullet *du jour* in U.S. health policy, but it still comprises a minority of the insurance market, and its ultimate impact and staying power are difficult to predict. After all, "revolutionary" changes in health care that were once much anticipated have, in retrospect, looked more like ill-fated fads. The future direction of market-led changes in the health system is consequently uncertain. We can, though, based on the history of American health care predict three dynamics with a high degree of confidence: first, issues of cost control will dominate the agenda for U.S. employers; second, there will be ongoing innovations in insurance products and experimentation with payment mechanisms that promise to address these problems; and third, these innovations will not resolve the cost issue and may exacerbate other problems (such as inequalities in access to health insurance).

In the political arena, there is now renewed interest—driven by the familiar combination of rising costs, eroding access, and economic insecurity—in health reform proposals that expand insurance coverage. These proposals have generally avoided the sheer ambition of the Clinton plan, abandoning both cost control and universal coverage as explicit goals in favor of an "ambitious incrementalism" that aims to cover around one-half to three-quarters of the uninsured population. The political calculus appears to be that health reform is more feasible if it extends coverage to the uninsured without imposing any mandates on employers, and without disturbing current arrangements for the already insured as well as for the insurance industry and health care providers. But rising federal budget deficits, a Congress polarized along party and ideological lines, and a political agenda dominated since 2001 by national security issues means that there is no easy path to health reform.

In the short term, there is a chance of adopting an incremental expansion of public insurance programs or tax credits, or some combination thereof. One compromise would enable the uninsured to use tax credits to buy group health insurance in the Federal Employees Health Benefits Program; individual mandate proposals that would make health insurance analogous to auto insurance also have attracted bipartisan attention. Or perhaps the newly enacted insurance expansion in Maine will prove to be a prelude to more state activism or even presage a template of federal funding made available for new state coverage initiatives.

The potential scope of any incremental expansions will be determined by the changing political and economic contexts, as well as developments in private health insurance. For example, the "buying down" of employer-sponsored private insurance through higher cost sharing and reduction of covered benefits could alter the calculus of health politics by intensifying middle-class anxieties about access to insurance, thereby creating an influential constituency for reform. The ongoing erosion of retiree health benefits, another fraying thread of the employer-based insurance system, could have a similar effect, especially as the baby boomers leave the workforce. There are other scenarios for change: the business community could decide that government action is necessary to save them from higher medical care costs or a political realignment could transform the legislative opportunities for comprehensive health reform.

Yet despite these possibilities it is not clear that health reform will move beyond (if it can get there) the limited steps of incrementalism, which would leave much of the uninsured population untouched and fall far short of universal coverage. Prospects for systemwide cost controls in the United States are even more remote. Although rising prescription drug prices may continue to draw political attention, there is currently little enthusiasm in the American polity for the type of global budget constraints that other nations' health systems employ.

Time and again over the last century, reformers have discovered new reasons why the enactment of universal coverage is imminent, only to be bitterly disappointed when reform turned out to be a mirage. The resilience of the status quo in American health policy should never be underestimated. The more things change in U.S. health policy, the more they seem to stay the same.

Notes

The author gratefully acknowledges the support of the Greenwall Foundation and Larry Churchill for his invaluable comments. I would also like to thank Kathy Griggs for her assistance in preparing this essay. The original essay has been revised for this edition.

1   Enthoven A, Kronick R. A consumer choice plan for the 1990s. *N Engl J Med* 1989; 320:29.
2   Woolhandler S, Campbell T, Himmelstein DU. Costs of health care administration in the United States and Canada. *N Engl J Med* 2003; 349:768–75.
3   Rublee D. Medical technology in Canada, Germany and the United States. *Health Aff (Millwood)* 1994; 13:113–7.
4   This paragraph draws on Bodenheimer TS, Grumbach K. *Understanding health policy.* Norwalk (CT): Appleton and Lange; 1995: 1–3.
5   US Census Bureau. *Health insurance coverage 2002.* Washington: The Bureau; 2003.
6   Burman LE, Uccello CE, Wheaton L, et al. *Tax subsidies for private health insurance.* Washington: Urban Institute; 2003. Available: http://www.urban.org/urlprint.cfm?ID= 8431 (Accessed 8 June 2004).
7   US Census Bureau. *Health insurance coverage 2002.* Washington: The Bureau; 2003.
8   Kaiser Commission on Medicaid and the Uninsured. *Health insurance coverage in America.* Washington: Kaiser Family Foundation; 2003.
9   Giled S, Lambew JM, Little S. *The growing share of uninsured workers employed by large firms.* New York: Commonwealth Fund; 2003.
10 Wysocki B, Zimmerman A. Wal-mart cost-cutting finds big target in health benefits. *Wall Street Journal* 2003 Sept 30; 1.
11 Kaiser Commission on Medicaid and the Uninsured. *Health insurance coverage in America.* Washington: Kaiser Family Foundation; 2003.
12 US Census Bureau. *Health insurance coverage 2002.* Washington: The Bureau; 2003.
13 Ayanian JZ, Weissman JS, Schneider EC, Ginsburg JA, Zaslavsky AM. Unmet health needs of uninsured adults in the United States. *JAMA* 2000; 284:2061–9.
14 Kaiser Commission on Medicaid and the Uninsured. *The uninsured and their access to health care.* Washington: Kaiser Family Foundation; 2001.
15 Ibid.
16 Institute of Medicine. *Care without coverage: too little, too late.* Washington: National Academy Press; 2002.

17 Crenshaw A. Study cites medical bills for many bankruptcies. *Washington Post* 2000 Apr 25; Sect E:1.

18 Himmelstein D, Woodhandler S. *Bleeding the patient: the consequences of corporate health care.* Monroe (ME): Common Courage Press; 2001: 24–5.

19 Kaiser Commission on Medicaid and the Uninsured. *Health insurance coverage in America.* Washington: Kaiser Family Foundation; 2003: 3.

20 US Congressional Budget Office. *The budget and economic outlook: fiscal years 2002–2011.* Washington: The Office; 2001.

21 Grumbach K. Insuring the uninsured: time to end the aura of invisibility. *JAMA* 2000; 284:214–6.

22 Leichter HM, editor. *Health policy reform in America: innovations from the states* (2nd ed.). Armonk (NY): M.E. Sharpe; 1997.

23 US Census Bureau. *Health insurance coverage 2002.* Washington: The Bureau; 2003.

24 Kaiser Commission on Medicaid and the Uninsured. *Out in the cold: enrollment freezes in six state children's health insurance programs withhold coverage from eligible children.* Washington: Kaiser Family Foundation; 2003: 1.

25 Ibid.

26 Feder J, Levitt L, O'Brien E, Rowland D. Covering the low income uninsured: the case for expanding public programs. *Health Aff (Millwood)* 2001; 20:27–39.

27 Kaiser Commission on Medicaid and the Uninsured. *Enrolling uninsured low-income children in Medicaid and CHIP.* Washington: Kaiser Family Foundation, 2002.

28 Kaiser Family Foundation. *Employer health benefits, 2003 annual survey.* Menlo Park (CA); 2003.

29 Oberlander J, Marmor TR. The path to universal health care. In: Borosage RL, Hickey R, eds. *The next agenda.* Boulder (CO): Westview Press; 2001: 93–125.

30 Deber R, Swan B. Canadian health expenditures: Where do we *really* stand internationally? *CMAJ* 1999; 160(12):1730–4.

31 Anderson GF, Hurst J, Hussey PS, Jee-Hughes M. Health spending and outcomes: trends in OECD countries, 1960–1998. *Health Aff (Millwood)* 2000; 19:150–7.

32 Gabel JR, Levitt L, Pickreign J, Whitmore H, Holve E, Hawkins S, et al. Job-based health insurance in 2000; premiums rise sharply while coverage grows. *Health Aff (Millwood)* 2000; 19(5):144–51.

33 Health Insurance Association of America. *Source book of health insurance data.* Washington: The Association; 1998.

34 Gabel JR, Ginsburg PB, Whitmore HH, Pickreign JD. Withering on the vine: the decline of indemnity health insurance. *Health Aff (Millwood)* 2000; 19(5):152–7.

35 Gabel JR. Ten ways HMOs have changed during the 1990s. *Health Aff (Millwood)* 1997; 16(3):134–45.

36 Kaiser Family Foundation. *Employer health benefits, 2003 annual survey chart pack.* Menlo Park (CA); 2003: 9.

37 Starr P. *The social transformation of American medicine.* New York: Basic; 1982.

38 Bodenheimer T. Physicians and the changing medical marketplace. *N Engl J Med* 1999; 340:585–8.

39 Levit K, Cowan C, Lazenby H, Sensening A, McDonnell P, Stiller J, et al. Health Spending in 1998: signals of change. *Health Aff (Millwood)* 2000; 19:124–32.

40 Deber R, Swan B. Canadian health expenditures: Where do we *really* stand internationally? *CMAJ* 1999; 160(12):1730–4.

41 Anderson GF, Hurst J, Hussey PS, Jee-Hughes M. Health spending and outcomes: trends in OECD countries, 1960–1998. *Health Aff (Millwood)* 2000; 19:150–7.

42 Center for Studying Health System Change. Tracking health care costs. Washington: 2003. Data Bulletin 25. Available: http://www.hschange.org/CONTENT/564/ (Accessed 2004 June 8).

43 Miller RH, Luft HS. Does managed care lead to better or worse quality of care? *Health Aff (Millwood)* 1997; 16:7–25.

44 Center for Studying Health System Change. Managed care pressures threaten access for the uninsured. Washington: 1999. Issue Brief 19. Available: http://www.hschange.org/CONTENT/62/?topic=topic02 (Accessed 2004 June 8).

45 Dudley RA, Luft HS. Managed care in transition. *N Engl J Med* 2001; 344:1087–92.

46 A patients' bill of rights for Canada? [editorial]. *CMAJ* 2001; 165(7):877.

47 Cauchi R. Managed care: where do we go from here? National Conference of State Legislatures; 1999. Available: http://www.ncsl.org/programs/pubs/399mancare.htm (Accessed 2004 June 8).

48 Robinson JC. The end of managed care. *JAMA* 2001; 285:2622–8.

49 Enthoven AC. Market forces and efficient health care systems. *Health Aff (Millwood)* 2004; 23:25.

50 Nichols LM, Ginsburg PB, Berenson RA, et al. Are market forces strong enough to deliver efficient health care systems? confidence is waning. *Health Aff (Millwood)* 2004; 23:13.

51 Ibid., 16.

52 Robinson JC. The end of managed care. *JAMA* 2001; 285:2622–8.

53 Reinhardt UE, Hussey PS, Anderson GF. U.S. health care spending in an international context. *Health Aff (Millwood)* 2004; 23:10.

54 Gabel J, Lo Sasso AT, Rice T. Consumer-driven health plans: are they more than talk now? *Health Aff 2002*; Web Exclusive: Available http://content.healthaffairs.org/cgi/content/full/hlthaff.w2.395v1/DC1 (Accessed 2004 June 8).

55 Fuchs VR. What's ahead for health insurance in the United States? *N Engl J Med* 2002; 346:1822–4.

56 Regopoulos LE, Trude S. Employers shift rising health care costs to workers: no long-term solution in sight. Center for Studying Health System Change; Washington: 2004. Issue Brief 83. Available: http://www.hschange.org/CONTENT/677/ (Accessed 2004 June 8).

57 Fuchs VR. What's ahead for health insurance in the United States? *N Engl J Med* 2002; 346:1822–4.

Wanted: A Clearly Articulated Social Ethic
for American Health Care
Uwe E. Reinhardt

Throughout the past three decades, Americans have been locked in a tenacious ideological debate whose essence can be distilled into the following pointed question: As a matter of national policy, and to the extent that a nation's health system can make it possible, should the child of a poor American family have the same chance of avoiding preventable illness or of being cured from a given illness as does the child of a rich American family?

The "yeas" in all other industrialized nations had won that debate hands down decades ago, and these nations have worked hard to put in place health insurance and health care systems to match that predominant sentiment. In the United States, on the other hand, the "nays" so far have carried the day. As a matter of conscious national policy, the United States always has and still does openly countenance the practice of rationing health care for millions of American children by their parents' ability to procure health insurance for the family or, if the family is uninsured, by their parents' willingness and ability to pay for health care out of their own pocket or, if the family is unable to pay, by the parents' willingness and ability to procure charity care in their role as health care beggars.

At any moment, over 40 million Americans find themselves without health insurance coverage, among them some 10 million children younger than 18 years. All available evidence suggests that this number will grow.[1] America's policy-making elite has remained unfazed by these statistics, reciting the soothing mantra that "to be uninsured in these United States does not means to be without care." There is, to be sure, some truth

Uwe E. Reinhardt, "Commentary—Wanted: A Clearly Articulated Social Ethic for American Health Care," from *Journal of the American Medical Association*, vol. 278, 1091–1096. © 1997 by the American Medical Association. Reprinted by permission of the publisher.

to the mantra. Critically ill, uninsured Americans of all ages usually receive adequate if untimely care under an informal, albeit unreliable, catastrophic health insurance program operated by hospitals and many physicians, largely on a voluntary basis. Under that informal program, hospitals and physicians effectively become insurance underwriters who provide succor to the hard-stricken uninsured and who extract the premium for that insurance through higher charges to paying patients. The alarming prospect is that the more effective the techniques of "managed care" will be in controlling the flow of revenue to physicians and hospitals, the more difficult it will be to play this insurance scheme, otherwise known as the "cost shift." It can be expected that, within the next decade, the growing number of the nation's uninsured will find themselves in increasingly dire straits.

But these straits have never been smooth for the uninsured, notwithstanding the soothing mantra cited earlier. Empirical research must have convinced policy makers long ago that our nation rations health care, health status, and life-years by ability to pay. It is known that other socioeconomic factors (such as income, family status, location, and so on) being equal, uninsured Americans receive, on average, only about 60% of the health services received by equally situated insured Americans.[2] This appears to be true even for the subgroup of adults whose health status is poor or only fair.[3] Studies have shown that uninsured Americans relying on the emergency departments of heavily crowded public hospitals experience very long waits before being seen by a physician, sometimes so long that they leave because they are too sick to wait any longer.[4-6] Studies have found that after careful statistical control for a host of socioeconomic and medical factors, uninsured Americans tend to die in hospitals from the same illness at up to triple the rate that is observed for equally situated insured Americans[7] and that, over the long run, uninsured Americans tend to die at an earlier age than do similarly situated insured Americans.[8] Indeed, before the managed care industry cut the fees paid physicians sufficiently to make fees paid by Medicaid look relatively attractive to physicians and hospitals, even patients insured by that program found it difficult to find access to timely care. In one study, in which research assistants approached private medical practices pretending to be Medicaid patients in need of care, 63% of them were denied access because the fees paid by Medicaid were then still paltry relative to the much higher fees from commercial insurers.[9]

If the champions of the uninsured believe that the assembly and dissemination of these statistics can move the nation's policy-making elite to embrace universal coverage, they may be in for a disappointment. Not only are the working majority of that elite unperturbed by these statistics, but they believe that rationing by price and ability to pay actually serves a greater national purpose. In that belief they find ample support in the writing of distinguished American academics. Commenting critically on the State Childrens' Health Insurance Program enacted by Congress in August 1997 as part of its overall budget bill, for example, Richard Epstein, author of the recently published *Mortal Peril: Our Inalienable Right to Health Care?*,[10] warns darkly that the new federal plan "introduces large deadweight administrative costs, invites overuse of medical care and reduces parental incentives to prevent accidents or illness." Summing up, he concludes: "We could do better with less regulation and less subsidy. *Scarcity matters, even in health care*" (italics added).[11]

Clearly, the scarcity Epstein would like to matter in health care would impinge much more heavily on the poor than it would on members of his own economic class, as Epstein surely is aware. In his view, by the way, Epstein finds distinguished company in former University of Chicago colleague Milton Friedman, the widely celebrated Nobel laureate in economics, who had proposed in 1991 that for the sake of economic efficiency, Medicare and Medicaid be abolished altogether and every American family have merely a catastrophic health insurance policy with a deductible of $20,000 per year or 30% of the previous two years' income, whichever is lower.[12] Certainly, Epstein and Friedman would be content to let price and family income ration the health care of American children. They rank prominently among the "nays."

In his book, Epstein frames the debate over the right to health care as a choice between the "maximization of social wealth" as a national objective and the "maximization of utility," by which he means human happiness. "Under wealth maximization," he writes, "individual preferences count only if they are backed by dollars. Preferences, however genuine, that are unmediated by wealth just do not count."[10(p32)] One implication of resource allocation with the objective of wealth maximization is that a physician visit to the healthy infant of a rich family is viewed as a more valuable activity than is a physician visit to the sick child of a poor family.[13] If one does not accept that relative valuation, then one does not favor wealth maximization as the binding social objective.

Although conceding that wealth maximization does imply a harsh algorithm for the allocation of scarce resources, Epstein nevertheless appears to embrace it, even for health care. Establishing positive legal rights to health care regardless of ability to pay, he argues, could well be counter-productive in the long run, because it detracts from the accumulation of wealth. "Allowing wealth to matter [in the allocation of health] is likely to do far better in the long run than any policy that insists on allocating health care without regard to ability to pay. To repeat, any effort to re-distribute from rich to poor in the present generation necessarily entails the redistribution from the future to the present generation."[13] Applying his proposition to the question posed at the outset of this commentary, the argument seems to be that poor children in one generation can prop-erly be left to suffer, so that all children of future generations may be made better off than they otherwise would have been.

One need not share Epstein's social ethic to agree with him that, over the long run, a nation that allocates resources generously to the unproduc-tive frail, whether rich or poor, is likely to register a relatively slower growth of material wealth than does a nation that is more parsimonious vis-à-vis the frail.[10(p114)] Nor does one need to share his social ethic to admire him for his courage to expose his conviction so boldly for open debate. Deep down, many members of this nation's policy-making elite, including many pundits who inspire that elite, and certainly a working majority of the Congress, share Epstein's view, although only rarely do they have the temerity to reveal their social ethic to public scrutiny. Although this school of thought may not hold a numerical majority in American society, they appear to hold powerful sway over the political process as it operates in this country.[14] In any event, they have for decades been able to preserve a status quo that keeps millions of American fami-lies uninsured, among them about 10 million children.

At the risk of violating the American taboo against class warfare, it is legitimate to observe that virtually everyone who shares Epstein's and Friedman's distributive ethic tends to be rather comfortably ensconced in the upper tiers of the nation's income distribution. Their prescriptions do not emanate from behind a Rawlsian[15] veil of ignorance concerning their own families' station in life. Furthermore, most well-to-do Americans who strongly oppose government-subsidized health insurance for low-income families and who see the need for rationing health care by price and ability to pay enjoy the full protection of government-subsidized, employer-provided, private health insurance that affords their families comprehensive coverage with out-of-pocket payments that are trivial relative to their own incomes and therefore spare their own families the pain of rationing altogether. The government subsidy in these policies flows from the regressive tax preference traditionally accorded employment-based health insurance in this country, whose premiums are paid out of pretax income.[16] This subsidy was estimated to have amounted to about $70 billion in 1991, of which 26% accrued to high-income households with annual incomes over $75,000.[17] The subsidy probably is closer to $100 billion now—much more than it would cost for every uninsured American to afford the type of coverage enjoyed by insured Americans. In fairness it must be stated that at least some critics of government-financed health insurance—Epstein among them—argue against this tax preference as well.[10(p182)] But that untoward tax preference has widespread supporters among members of Congress of all political stripes, and also in the executive suites of corporate America.

This regressive tax preference would only be enlarged further under the medical savings accounts (MSAs) now favored by organized American medicine. Under that concept, families would purchase catastrophic health insurance policies with annual deductibles of $3,000 to $5,000 per family, and they would finance their deductible out of MSAs into which they could deposit $3,000 to $5,000 per year out of the family's pretax income. In terms of absolute, after-tax dollars, this construct effectively would make the out-of-pocket cost of a medical procedure much lower for high-income families (in high marginal tax brackets) than it would for low-income families. It is surely remarkable to see such steadfast support in the Congress for this subsidy for the well-to-do, in a nation that claims to lack the resources to afford every mother and child the peace of mind and the health benefits that come with universal health insurance, a privilege mothers and children in other countries have long taken for granted. Unwittingly, perhaps, by favoring this regressive scheme to finance health care, physicians take a distinct stand on the preferred distributive ethic for American health care. After all, can it be doubted that the MSA construct would lead to rationing childrens' health care by income class?

Typically, the opponents of universal health insurance cloak their sentiments in actuarial technicalities or in the mellifluous language of the standard economic theory of markets,[18] thereby avoiding a debate on ideology that truly might engage the public. It is time, after so many decades, that the rival factions in America's policy-making elite debate openly their distinct visions of distributive ethic for health care in this country, so that the general public can decide by which of the rival elites it wishes to be ruled. A good start in that debate could be made by answering forthrightly the pointed question posed at the outset.

Notes

1   Thorpe KE. *The Rising Number of Uninsured Workers: An Approaching Crisis in Health Care Financing.* Washington, DC: The National Coalition on Health Care; September 1997.

2   *Behavioral Assumptions for Estimating the Effects of Health Care Proposals.* Washington, DC: Congressional Budget Office; November 1993; Table 3:viii.

3   Long SH, Marquis MS. *Universal Health Insurance and Uninsured People: Effects on Use and Costs: Report to Congress.* Washington, DC: Office of Technology Assessment and Congressional Research Service, Library of Congress; August 5, 1994; Figure 1:4.

4   Kellerman AL. Too sick to wait. *JAMA.* 1991; 266: 1123–1124.

5   Baker DW, Stevens CD, Brook RH. Patients who leave a public hospital emergency department without being seen by a physician. *JAMA.* 1991; 266: 1085–1090.

6   Bindman AB, Grumbach K, Keane D, Rauch L, Luce JM. Consequences of queuing for care at a public hospital emergency department. *JAMA.*1991; 266: 1091–1096.

7   Hadley J, Steinberg EP, Feder J. Comparison of uninsured and privately insured hospital patients. *JAMA.* 1991; 265: 374–379.

8   Franks P, Clancy CM, Gold MR. Health insurance and mortality: evidence from a national cohort. *JAMA.* 1993; 270: 737–741.

9   The ultimate denial: rationing is a reality. *Issue Scan: Q Rep Health Care Issues Trends from Searle.* 1994; 4(2): 5.

10 Epstein RA. *Mortal Peril: Our Inalienable Right to Health Care?* New York, NY: Addison-Wesley; 1997.

11 Epstein RA. Letter to the editor. *The New York Times.* August 10, 1997: 14.

12 Friedman M. Gammon's law points to health care solution. *The Wall Street Journal.* November 12, 1991: A19.

13 Reinhardt UE. Abstracting from distributional effects, this policy is efficient. In: Barer M, Getzen T, Stoddard G, eds. *Health, Health Care, and Health Economics: Perspectives on Distribution.* London, England: John Wiley & Sons Ltd; 1997: 1–53.

14 Taylor H, Reinhardt UE. Does the system fit? *Health Manage Q.* 1991; 13(3): 2–10.

15 Rawls J. *A Theory of Justice.* Cambridge, Mass: Harvard University Press; 1971.

16 Reinhardt UE. Reorganizing the financial flows in American health care. *Health Aff (Millwood).* 1993; 12(suppl): 172–193.

17 Butler SM. A policymaker's guide to the health care crisis, I. *Heritage Talking Points.* Washington, DC: The Heritage Foundation: February 12, 1992: 5.

18 Reinhardt UE. Economics. *JAMA.* 1996; 275: 1802–1804.

From Bismarck to Medicare—A Brief History of Medical Care Payment in America

Donald L. Madison

At the outset, a word of explanation. This discursive essay borrows its title from a more focused one, written over 60 years ago by the distinguished historian Henry Sigerist, who titled his study of the original social insurance program, "From Bismarck to Beveridge."[1]

In the same way that certain scientific phenomena demand attention to genesis and change over time (meteorology, embryology and pathology come to mind), so does the study of contemporary social policy require that one know something of its past. The present essay reflects this view.[2] It is meant to serve as an accessible introduction—for students and other beginners—to health insurance in America and related matters; but I have written it as a history, not as an explanatory manual.

I have inserted here and there—wherever they seemed to fit best within the story—a few "asides" to explain terms and concepts that may be unfamiliar, or to clarify words and phrases that the reader will have heard before but that are sometimes misunderstood.

Any chronological narrative on this topic must either reach or anticipate the interface between past and present. I have elected to anticipate it and will end with the enactment and implementation of America's most important insurance program—Medicare. Much has occurred since July 1966, when Medicare began (it was enacted a year earlier). Yet, most of this post-Medicare activity has consisted either of unsuccessful schemes to expand financial access or of similarly unsuccessful—or temporarily successful—attempts to curb the escalating costs of health services. I shall not attempt to account for all the tactics that the various "players" have used except to say that most of them came from the private sector; relatively few were legislated remedies. All of these schemes had names, or acronyms, which those involved once knew and may still remember. While it is certainly useful to know the terminology of the moment, it is less important to remember, for example, what a PSRO was. The constantly changing world of "managed care" is likewise outside the scope of this essay, as are the details of the grandly proposed but ultimately failed Clinton health plan. I justify these omissions with the observation that the conceptual antecedents (though not the details) of virtually every scheme being pushed toward or likely to be proposed in the near future, were already in place prior to the enactment of Medicare.

Of course, the political debate over health care financing continues. It includes both the seemingly eternal issue of cost containment and the more pressing question of how to cover those Americans who are without protection. But here I will stick to history and leave these important but yet unanswered questions to other, more presentist commentators.

The Basis of Health Insurance

Medical care is, among other things, a service for sale. It costs something to produce and to purchase. How the money flows is the stuff of medical care financing.

Once upon a time paying for medical care was a simple matter. Doctors treated patients, and in return patients paid the doctor's fee *at the time of illness.* That's all there was to it. The fee covered nearly everything. Hospitals were not a part of the picture; pharmacies were, but not nearly so much nor so often as now. There were no diagnostic centers or commercial laboratories. If the patient ran short of funds to pay the doctor, barter was often accepted, since the doctor's costs consisted mostly of his time and household expenses. The office, with no staff beyond the doctor himself and his wife, was part of the home.[3] No longer. Office lease, malpractice insurance, equipment purchase and maintenance, corporate taxes, medical supplies, continuing education, automobile depreciation, professional society dues, reference lab fees, staff salaries with social security payments and other fringe benefits, debt service, and so on, ad infinitum, must all now be paid as the necessary costs of carrying on a medical practice. A chicken, a bushel of apples, or a new fence in lieu of a fee doesn't help much in meeting these kinds of costs.

Still, the physician's side of medical care financing is actually simple compared to the patient's. Hospital costs now consume roughly 35% of the medical care dollar.[4] In addition to the basic charge, usually calculated as for a hotel on a per day basis, payments must be made for laboratory, radiography, and electrocardiography charges (including the fees of the medical specialists who interpret each of these three technological forms of diagnosis), procedures of all sorts, emergency room fees, operating room charges, anesthesiologist's fees, pathologist's fees, clinical consultations, drugs, supplies and appliances. (The average total charge now exceeds $1,500 per day in many urban hospitals.) Then there are the costs of prescription drugs, nursing homes, home care, and so on. And this doesn't consider the *indirect* costs to the patient (such as transportation or child care) or the *opportunity* costs (such as income foregone due to time away from work).

Obviously, even a moderately severe episode of sickness today can leave all but the most wealthy patient unable to pay *at the time the medical care is needed.* Actually, that has been true for a long time, and it is why the old method of paying at the time of illness had to be replaced by the idea of collective financing—the regular collection of small amounts of money from everyone to pay for the care of people who are sick. In this way, people could be protected (insured) from financial ruin caused by the unpredictability of illness. They agreed to absorb a *small certain loss* (the known amount of the premium) to avoid a *large uncertain loss* (the unknown but probably large outlay for medical and hospital care, if and when it was required).

There are two main kinds of health insurance at work in the United States: *social insurance* and *private insurance.* Most of this essay will explain the evolution and some of the features and variations of these two. Social insurance came first.

Before I summarize the history of social insurance I should explain what it is. The distinctive characteristic of social insurance as compared to private insurance is its compulsory nature. The government requires coverage by law. It may provide the insurance itself, or it may require (or allow) people to obtain it in the private sector. The best-known American example of social insurance is Old Age, Survivors, Disability and Health Insurance, usually called, simply, Social Security. It includes a social *health* insurance program, Medicare. Social Security is a federal program. At the state level, probably the most familiar example of social insurance (with indirect health care benefits) is the liability insurance that all states require automobile owners to purchase.

Social insurance is distinguished from *public assistance* by the payment of premiums that bear some relation to benefits—the majority of social insurance in the United States is financed through equal employer and employee contributions held in the Social Security Trust Fund—and by the principle that benefits are given to the recipients as a matter of right, not as charity. *Public assistance* is *not* insurance; it is paid for out of general tax revenue to people found to be in need, regardless of how much if anything they paid in taxes. Of the two major government medical care financing programs in the United States, one, Medicare, is social insurance; the other, Medicaid, is public assistance. A large number of government programs provide health benefits, but only two of these (Medicare and Workers' Compensation) are social insurance.

Social Insurance: Bismarck (1883)

Insurance for the *indirect costs of illness* came into being well before insurance for the *direct costs of medical care.* Before the 20th century, few hospitals charged patients anything. Physicians did charge fees, of course, but except for surgical operations, these were usually modest; the doctor wouldn't have been able to collect otherwise. But when a workman fell ill his family faced a more basic problem—the loss of the breadwinner's income. There was no such thing yet as unemployment insurance or sick leave.

To meet the problem of income lost because of sickness, workers organized their own mutual benefit funds, usually through their social clubs, lodges, or "friendly societies." These workers' clubs collected small, regular payments from each member. Then, when a member fell ill and was unable to work, the fund helped out. The other time when the friendly society helped was when a worker died. The family received a modest cash benefit to help with the expense of the burial.

These workers' mutual benefit societies had existed in Europe since the 13th century, but their growth accelerated during the last half of the 19th century, when the industrial revolution and accompanying urbanization produced both a greater concentration of workers and greater risk of illness and injury. Along with urban industrialization came labor unrest, which led to political agitation.

In the new nation-state of Germany, Prince Otto Eduard Leopold von Bismarck, the "Iron Chancellor," was in firm control. Bismarck was disturbed, however, by the rapid gains the socialists were making among the German industrial workers. Despite his suppressive antisocialism law of

1878, the popularity of socialism as an idea continued to grow. So, in 1883 Bismarck changed tactics. He reasoned that a generous, paternalistic state might win the workers' loyalties, or at least mollify those that were the most discontented. That was why he proposed a social insurance program that would be operated and directly financed by the state: he wanted it to be closely identified with his government.

But Bismarck hadn't counted on the strength of the mutual benefit societies. By 1883 there were many of these sickness funds—called, in German, *Krankenkassen*—and the workers had a vested interest in them. And this, combined with a certain distaste, shared by workers and employers alike, for Prussian-style government administration, convinced Bismarck that it would be politically expedient to alter his original plan. So instead of getting the state-run program he had wanted, Bismarck settled for a state-*mandated* system in which the German government would require all industrial workers to join one of these employment-based (operated either by the workers or the employer) *private* sickness funds.

Students have sometimes asked after hearing this description: "Was Bismarck the father of socialized medicine?" My response is that "Bismarck would not have been pleased with your question if by 'socialized medicine' you mean *socialist* medicine, since Bismarck was antisocialist."

This is probably a good place to begin defining terms, starting with that one. "Socialized medicine" is a phrase without specific meaning; it has been (and still is) used mainly by those who are unwilling or unable to be more precise. Physicians have also used these two words pejoratively in referring to some greater degree of organization of and/or control over medical practice than they would prefer. They have applied the term "socialized medicine" at various times to Blue Cross, well baby clinics in public health departments, salaried employment of physicians by hospitals, medical faculty practice plans, Medicare, the medical care system of the former Soviet Union, the British National Health Service, neighborhood health centers for the poor, publicly administered mass immunization for polio, Veterans Administration hospitals, public campaigns against venereal disease, government payment for medical services under the "Crippled Children" program, HMOs, PPOs, and student health services at universities. Clearly, as times change, so do the applications of the term. Politicians and public relations consultants have also used it whenever the connotation of socialism served their purpose. It should be apparent from the above that the phrase "socialized medicine" has no place in the lexicon of medical care financing.

If Bismarck was not the father of "socialized medicine," was he then the father of social insurance? Yes, the 1883 German social insurance program was the world's first. Soon other European nations began following Bismarck's example, although not for the same political reasons.

Social Insurance: Lloyd George (1911)

Great Britain was one of the nations to follow the German example. Under the leadership of David Lloyd George, the chancellor of the Exchequer (the British name for secretary of the Treasury), Britain enacted a national program of social insurance in 1911. Because Lloyd George preferred the word "health" to "sickness," it was called the National *Health* Insurance Act. Like the German model, the British program was also based on preexisting mutual benefit funds (called in Britain "friendly societies"). And like Bismarck's program, British health insurance covered only manual workers, and not their dependents.

These two major programs were early examples of *national health insurance.* Since that is a term you will hear often, this is a good time to define it. It refers to a national program of social insurance that finances medical care for all or part of the population. Usually the term is used for programs that cover *most* of a country's population (like, for example, approximately two-thirds in the Netherlands, more than 85% in Belgium and Germany, and virtually everyone in Canada). It is no longer, as in Lloyd George's day, used to describe compulsory social insurance programs that cover only industrial workers or some other minority of the citizens of a country (for example, the approximately 15% of Americans aged 65 and older who are covered by Medicare). Under national health insurance, the government, acting either directly or through private sector agents, makes payments to physicians, hospitals, pharmacies, laboratories, and so on, which themselves operate privately. However, in order to participate in the program these private entities must meet certain standards that have been set by the national insurance plan.

Both the German and the British national health insurance programs (and the others that were enacted before World War I) primarily paid cash benefits at the time of sickness and a burial benefit at death. It is also true that these programs paid for physicians' services, but this benefit was, at least in the beginning, less important.

The practice of mutual benefit societies paying for physicians' services came about gradually. Originally these societies' sickness funds didn't involve doctors at all. But soon the age-old question arose: how could a friendly society be certain that the beneficiary was actually sick and deserving of the cash benefit, and not merely malingering? That's when doctors entered the picture. For a sum that varied with the size of the benefit society (so much per member per year) a doctor would agree to examine and certify each case of illness. The main reason for paying the doctor by "capitation" instead of some other method—fee-for-service, for example—was that capitation was so much easier for these small, worker-run funds to administer.

Then, since it was obviously in the interest of the mutual benefit society to restore the sick member to health as rapidly as possible, to minimize the drain on the fund, *treatment* was added to the doctor's original job of *certifying.* And the doctor usually also contracted to furnish whatever medicine the sick member might need. So by the time of the early national health insurance laws, physicians' services rendered in the "surgery" (office) and in the homes of patients, were already among the benefits that most German Krankenkassen and British friendly societies were providing their members.

The German program was extended little by little until by the 1920s it covered virtually everyone. By contrast, British national health insurance was never extended beyond its original target, the industrial workers—not even to their dependents. Universal coverage for Britons came only after World War II, when in 1948 a new Labor government replaced Lloyd George's original program of national health insurance with a *national health service.*

The distinction between those two terms—"national health *insurance*" and "national health *service*"—is often confusing. The difference is this: In a *national health insurance* program, government controls the financing only, while in a *national health service*, the government controls *both* the financing *and* the delivery of services. In a national health service the government (though not necessarily the *national* government) employs many of the physicians, as well as the other health personnel, and it operates the clinics and hospitals. This arrangement is often modified, as in the United Kingdom, where the medical specialists are government employees but the general practitioners are not. (Although almost all British GPs are exclusive contractors with the National Health Service, they are actually in private practice.) The Scandinavian countries and Finland have both a national health service *and* a national health insurance program. In these countries local government runs the hospitals and health centers and employs those physicians who are not in private practice, but the national government also operates a health insurance scheme, which helps pay for the care delivered by the government-operated centers and hospitals as well as that delivered by private practitioners.

The First American Campaign: Social Insurance and the AMA (1912–1920)

The year after Lloyd George's British program was enacted a group of American social welfare activists began planning a similar sickness insurance program for industrial workers in the United States. The American Association for Labor Legislation (AALL) had already led a successful effort to enact workmen's compensation laws, and when it turned its attention to health insurance the group followed the same strategy it had used in that earlier campaign: first, draft a model law, and then try to get it enacted by as many state legislatures as possible.

At the outset, this first American push for social health insurance appeared promising. Launched in the wake of the British program's success, it was also riding on the favorable momentum of other Progressive era social reforms. Further, in 1916 the AALL gained an important ally when the American Medical Association lent its support to the campaign, appointing a study committee and even assigning one of its staff to work full-time in the AALL's New York headquarters. But ultimately, the AALL proposal went nowhere. A few states appointed study commissions, and only one, New York, actually introduced it as legislation.[5]

It failed for a combination of reasons—first and most important bad timing. World War I marked a watershed in American political opinion. With the war the Progressive era was over, and states became less interested in enacting social legislation. Social insurance, which after all had been a German invention (Germany was the enemy), fell out of favor. Yet the AALL's health insurance plan may have been doomed anyway, since most of big business as well as some of the most important labor leaders opposed it. Like the British program, the American proposal would have required employers to insure industrial workers for sick leave and the costs of physicians' services. It would also have paid a small burial benefit, a feature that raised the ire of the life insurance companies.

And although the leadership of the AMA had generally favored health insurance, the association's grassroots membership, which had been ambivalent at best, turned adamantly against it after the war. Speaking to a county medical society meeting in 1919, one New York physician called the AALL plan "Un-American, Unsafe, Uneconomic, Unscientific, Unfair and Unscrupulous," the invention of "Paid Professional Philanthropists, busybody Social Workers, Misguided Clergymen, and Hysterical women."[6] In 1920 the AMA House of Delegates made a dramatic and permanent about face. It repudiated those of its leaders who had supported the AALL's health insurance proposal and declared its opposition henceforth to "any plan embodying the system of compulsory contributory insurance against illness, or any other plan . . . provided, controlled, or regulated by any state or the Federal Government."[7]

The AMA's leaders made an important discovery in 1920. They discovered the association's membership base—what it stood for and, more important, what it stood against. To use a metaphor from immunology, the AALL episode had an antigenic effect on the AMA. Afterward, every time a government-sponsored or even a local, consumer-sponsored health plan was suggested—any program that the doctors themselves did not control—organized medicine's antibody titer rose sharply.

Sheppard-Towner and Federal Grant Programs
(1921 and Beyond)

Health insurance as a public issue went into hibernation in the United States during the 1920s and would not be raised again seriously for another 20 years. This isn't to say that nothing of significance happened in American medical care before the 1940s. Actually, quite a lot happened. In 1921 Congress enacted the first *federal grant program* to assist the delivery of public health services, the Sheppard-Towner Act.

Under Sheppard-Towner the federal government gave matching money to the states to be used for health instruction and preventive care for mothers and children from poor families; the money also helped purchase and deliver fresh milk for babies. The passage by Congress of Sheppard-Towner was an indirect result of the 19th (suffrage) Amendment (1920): congressmen feared the women's vote, and they saw Sheppard-Towner as a women's program. The AMA, its antibody titer still running high in the wake of the AALL episode, opposed the Sheppard-Towner Act when it was introduced and continued to oppose it throughout the 1920s. Finally, in 1929, the AMA's lobbying paid off. When the authorization had to be extended, Congress and President Hoover allowed Sheppard-Towner to expire.

The story of Sheppard-Towner is interesting not just for the political dynamics; it was the first American example of using a federal grant program for a health purpose—and the *grant program* is yet another way (other than out-of-pocket payment, insurance, and welfare) by which health services may be financed. Today, when the central government wishes to transfer funds to the local level for some special purpose, it is likely to do it via a grant program. In the United States almost all public health services at the local level are supported partly by what are called "formula grants" (matching grants given by the federal government to each state according to a formula that considers the size of the state's population, the relative income level of its citizens, and other indicators of need). This was the way in which the money for Sheppard-Towner was distributed. But the federal government now also makes what are called "project" grants, awarded in response to competitive proposals received from not-for-profit organizations of various kinds (e.g., local government, universities, research institutes, nonprofit community organizations). The federal government funds a wide array of health resources and services via project grants. Their purposes include biomedical research, residency training in primary care, and, in the area of medical care, operation of community health centers in underserved rural and urban locations.

Paying Hospitals and Doctors (1900 and Beyond)

The reason I've said almost nothing thus far about private health insurance is that there wasn't any—or hardly any. A few lodges in urban locations contracted with a doctor to care for their members (the American equivalent of the British friendly societies).[8] And during the last half of the 19th century some commercial life insurance companies branched out to offer accident insurance, so that if a workman lost an arm or a leg and had purchased this kind of insurance he could collect the amount stated in the policy. Also, by about 1915 most states were requiring employers to carry workmen's compensation insurance, which meant that if a worker was injured on the job the employer's insurance would pay for lost wages and for medical care associated with the injury. Workmen's compensation insurance was private insurance, but it was a public law that mandated that the employer carry it.

That was pretty much all there was in the private sector—except for the many industrial firms that provided medical care on the job and the very few that also cared for employees and dependents for non-job-related illnesses.[9] Both of these exceptions were employment-related, but neither represented insurance; that is, the companies delivered the medical care directly and provided it free (or at a low charge) to their employees as a part of the work environment. Other than this, there was essentially no collective financing of medical care in America—public or private—before the 1930s. Earlier it hadn't been necessary, and in the 1920s, by which time it was necessary, there were still no organizational arrangements in place.

Before the 20th century people didn't go to hospitals if they could be cared for at home. And when they were hospitalized they were seldom charged, since the public saw the hospitals—and the hospitals saw themselves—as charities. Gradually that changed. Hospitals became more essential to medical practice, more complex, and much more expensive to operate, until by the early 1920s most of them were charging any patient who could pay. This change brought a new social problem for which there appeared to be no easy solution: a family's financial resources were now endangered not only by the unpredictable indirect *costs of sickness*, but also by the unpredictable direct *expenses of medical care*.

The medical care cost issue had two parts: one was the hospital charge; the other was the doctor's charge. Too many doctors' fees seemed excessively high, and with no apparent justification. The problem related to the way doctors set their fees. Medical writers on this topic generally agreed that each doctor should be left to determine the proper fee for his service and that it ought to be based on three considerations:

1. *The relative skill and standing of the physician.* Established physicians, like established lawyers, could justifiably charge more than novices and those with less standing in the community. Also, those who called themselves specialists could charge more.[10]

2. *The nature of the service.* Not only did surgery obviously require a certain technical proficiency, it could also demonstrate a rather immediate and dramatic result. Moreover, it carried some risk. Accordingly, operations should command high fees.

3. *The ability of the patient to pay.* The physician's ability to judge the economic standing of his patient was still in the 1920s considered part of the art of medical practice. The 1922 "Crowning Edition" of the leading textbook on practice economics, Cathell's *Book on the Physician Himself*, advised physicians: "while the grocer may charge every customer the same for a pound of sugar, the physician cannot do this and must have a sliding scale of charges according to the class of society to which the

patient belongs." Two problems that writers in the popular press complained about throughout the 20s was that physicians often erred in judging the class of society to which a patient belonged, and that their "sliding scale of charges" seemed always to be sliding up.

Cathell had *fee-for-service* in mind when offering his advice about the "sliding scale." Yet fee-for-service was only one of three traditional ways in which physicians were remunerated. All three are as old as the profession itself, and each has variations and combinations. For example, one very old variation of fee-for-service is *case-payment* (the physician receives a fixed sum for giving a patient all necessary care for a particular illness or condition, e.g., pregnancy).

It is important when thinking about remuneration to separate how the *patient* pays (and thus how the *practice as an organization* is financed) from how the *individual physician* is paid. Note in this respect the two-part definitions below for "capitation" and "fee-for-service."

> Capitation is (1) a method of financing medical *practice.* The *practice* receives—from an insurance company, health maintenance organization, employer, membership association, university, or government— a fixed amount for each person (a "per capita" amount) who is enrolled, subscribed, registered, or otherwise entitled to receive medical care from the practice. This fixed amount is paid whether the person actually uses the service or not, and regardless of how much service he or she uses. The amount of the capitation payment is negotiated in advance between the practice and some health care financing agency. In the United States, many medical practices are financed partly by capitation, and a few large multispecialty group practices are financed entirely by this method. Capitation is also (2) a method of remunerating *physicians.* This method of physician payment, which is nearly as old as fee-for-service and salary, does not exist in its pure form in the United States. (Note that medical groups receiving capitation payments do *not* compensate their individual physician members by this method. Also, those primary care physicians who are paid by managed care organizations on a capitation basis will usually see many more patients who are not members of the managed care organization and who pay on a fee-for-service basis.) A good example of capitation as a means of remunerating individual physicians is the British National Health Service, where general practitioners receive a fixed amount for each person on their "list." (Specialists in the British National Health

Service are salaried.) General practitioners in several other European countries also receive much of their remuneration in the form of capitation payments.

Salary is another common method of paying physicians—and it is one of the two most common methods for paying other health care workers (the other being the hourly wage). The level of the physician's salary may be fixed relative to training, specialty, seniority, merit, time spent in the practice, or any number of other considerations, but it is *not directly* related to the amount of money the physician generates or the number of patients served. Note again: the *physician* may be paid via fixed salary regardless of whether the *practice* is financed by fee-for-service, capitation, contract, budget appropriation, or any other method.

Fee-for-service is (1) a common method of financing medical *practice*. Under fee-for-service the *practice* sells its services (physician visits, procedures, lab tests, etc.) to patients, who pay (or have paid on their behalf) a fee for each individual "service" that the practice provides or supplies. Fee-for-service is also (2) a method of remunerating individual *physicians*. The *physician* is paid with (or in proportion to) the fees he or she generates. Note: physicians who work in fee-for-service *practices* may or may not be remunerated themselves on a fee-for-service basis. They may, in fact, receive a fixed salary, or a formula share of practice income, or even (rarely) a per capita amount as the basis of their individual payment. In other words, fee-for-service *financing*—of the practice—is distinct from fee-for-service *remuneration*—of the physician.

Each of these three methods for paying physicians has its protagonists and critics.

Capitation is especially popular among those who must pay the bills. When the amount of money that will change hands is fixed and known in advance, fiscal planning and the control of expenditures are easier. Also, when the physician's responsibility for providing the patient's care is absolute, and not discretionary, he or she is much more likely to act according to the patient's need for care, and not according to the physician's ability to collect the fee or the patient's ability to pay it. In fact, one of the more important advantages claimed for capitation is that the physician need never worry about the patient's ability to pay for whatever care is needed, since it has in effect already been paid for. "Whatever care is needed" includes, of course, sending the patient to other physicians for referrals and consultations, something fee-for-service physicians have at times been reluctant to do for fear of losing patients to competitors.

The critics of capitation say that the physician who is remunerated in this way has an incentive to do as little as possible for the patient since the amount of payment will be the same no matter what. Capitation's defenders reply that such scrimping, if done very often, would offend the patient, who would then change his or her "enrollment" to another practice (or another "plan") and perhaps persuade others to do likewise, thereby causing, ultimately, a far greater loss of income to the offending physician.

Salary, it is claimed by its detractors, best suits physicians who are lazy, since the salary carries no financial incentive toward either individual productivity or quality. Its defenders reply to the contrary that the salaried physician's disincentives to skimp or cut corners are in fact great, since under salary it is not one's volume of fees (as with fee-for-service) or the size of one's practice (as with capitation) that may be jeopardized by poor performance, but one's very employment. Further, they point out that some of the most reputable and prestigious practice organizations— private, academic, and governmental—remunerate their physicians by salary.

Fee-for-service can deliver, at least potentially, the largest income to the physician, and this may partially explain its popularity among the medical profession. (It may also yield, potentially, the lowest income.) Moreover, its defenders say, the fee-for-service method of payment rewards the physician who works hardest. As with any other piecework method, those who work the most (ergo, who presumably are the most deserving) are remunerated with the most. There is evidence that office-based doctors work longer hours and see more patients when they are paid on a fee-for-service basis than when they are on salary.

There has also been much criticism of fee-for-service. Virtually all of it is directed in one way or another to the basic incentive that is at work whenever physicians sell their services in exchange for fees. George Bernard Shaw said it this way:

> That any sane nation, having observed that you could provide for the supply of bread by giving bakers a pecuniary interest in baking for you, should go on to give a surgeon a pecuniary interest in cutting off your leg, is enough to make one despair of political humanity. But

that is precisely what we have done. And the more appalling the mutilation, the more the mutilator is paid. He who corrects the ingrowing toe-nail receives a few shillings; he who cuts your inside out receives hundreds of guineas.[11]

Shaw's surgical examples, especially his fascination with surgical "mutilation," may seem old-fashioned to us now, but the principle applies still. Fee-for-service is indeed an inducement for the physician to favor the more highly remunerative procedures over the lower paying services (such as listening and explaining). There is ample evidence that the incentive for the physician to do a "greater" service when a higher fee is linked to it works very well.

Private doctors in the United States have generally believed that fee-for-service is the most advantageous for them, the most amenable to their control, and the most difficult for government or private purchasers of care to manipulate. However, health care planners and financing sources (including employers, unions, managed care firms and government) dislike the open-endedness of fee-for-service and the difficulty it presents for controlling expenditures. Yet, because the two payment methods that are fixed (capitation and salary) allow such "third parties" greater potential control over the amount of physicians' future remuneration, private doctors are wary of these methods. They believe, no doubt correctly, that in the event of a fiscal crisis such control would be used. On the other hand, some observers believe that the greatest threat to the fiscal stability of the "third parties" is the lack of control over expenditures that has long been associated with fee-for-service.

Indemnity Insurance and "Moral Hazard" (1900–1940)

Historically, there have been *three main types* of private health "insurance" in the United States: (1) *indemnity insurance*, (2) *service benefit plans*, and (3) *direct service plans*. All of our present-day health care financing mechanisms are derived from these three.

Only one of the three types—indemnity insurance—is true insurance by the traditional meaning of that term. The insurance principle holds that in exchange for regular payment of the premium, the insurance company will compensate the insured the amount of a loss ("indemnification"). This is easy to understand if the loss was caused by theft or fire or death, since these "indemnities" are easy to recognize, and the amount of each of them is known (it was stated in the policy in advance). In the case of health insurance, however, the exact nature and therefore the amount of the "indemnity" aren't as clear. Who is to say what is an illness? And who is to say how much or what kind of medical attention is necessary? In fact, for a long time most commercial insurance companies refused to write policies against the cost of medical care because it was so unpredictable. When they finally did begin selling health insurance on a larger scale at the end of the 1930s, the commercial insurers placed strict limits on the amounts they would pay, and they demanded to see the bill (showing what the patient had been charged by the doctor or the hospital) as proof that the policy holder did indeed have an "indemnity" before they would pay (the amount of the bill up to the limit stated in the policy). Since indemnity insurance was strictly a matter between the insurance company and the policyholder, the doctor (and hospital) could charge the patient whatever they wished. The patient paid the bill; the patient submitted the claim; the patient received the check back from the insurance company; while the doctor did nothing. This series of events explains why the medical profession has long favored indemnity insurance: in its pure form it doesn't involve doctors at all. Nor does it place any restrictions on patients, such as telling them which doctors they may or may not use.

The private health insurance industry didn't really come on the scene until the 1930s. Why so late? Other kinds of commercial insurance had been available for a long time. Insurance companies did a good business selling casualty insurance, life insurance, and so on.[12] But they steered clear of health insurance.

The main reason was something they called "moral hazard." One of the guiding principles of the insurance business is to protect the carrier against it. I never quite understood what "moral hazard" was until I asked an economist friend to explain it to me. He told his story: It seems that a house had burned to the ground, and some of the neighbors suspect the owner of knowing more than he is willing to admit about the fire's cause. One day the owner's best friend asks him to reveal, confidentially, how the fire started.

"Friction," the owner says.

"I don't understand," the friend replies. "What kind of friction could cause a house to burn down?"

The owner smiles: "The friction of a $30,000 house rubbing against a $90,000 insurance policy."

That's moral hazard. It's the question of whether there exists even a remote possibility that the insurance policy could have caused the loss. That possibility represents the moral hazard.

There is a moral hazard problem with any kind of insurance, but it is reduced in the case of life insurance by a law that exacts a harsh punishment for committing murder. Likewise, the law against arson reduces the moral hazard for fire insurance.

But what about health insurance? The early commercial insurers found that with health insurance the moral hazard question was much more complicated. It had to do with the insurance company's inability to know what the real need for the service was. How could one ever know this, for sure, when the party being paid (ultimately) from the insurance for having rendered a service was the same party that declared the service necessary? Even more, how could one trust that the indemnity was real and accurate when the party receiving payment was the same one who (1) discovered the problem, (2) decided *which* services were called for, and (3) set the price for those services? When the service was medical care, how can one be confident that it was not delivered because the doctor knew that the patient had an insurance policy? Insurance companies could easily see that the moral hazard question made insuring for medical care much different, and more difficult, than insuring a house against fire or a life against death. So they generally avoided health insurance.

Service Benefit Plans and the Birth of the Blues
(1929–1945)

The American private health insurance industry got under way during the Great Depression. This was a time when people had little money to pay hospitals, which left many private hospitals with unpaid bills and empty beds (while at the same time public hospitals, supported by tax dollars to care for those unable to pay, were operating at full capacity). Not surprisingly, the initiative came from the hospitals, which had been experiencing collection problems throughout the 1920s.

In 1929, a private hospital in Dallas, Texas, came up with a plan that it thought would help it financially. The Baylor University Hospital approached the Dallas public school teachers with a proposal: if the teachers would allow a small amount (50 cents) to be deducted from their monthly paychecks and turned over to the Baylor Hospital, the hospital would in return provide up to 21 days of hospitalization each year for any teacher who needed it. The teachers consented to this novel plan, which worked so well that other hospitals in Dallas, and soon elsewhere around the country, began imitating it.

This was, of course, not "insurance" by the customary meaning. The plan did not indemnify its subscribers for a loss; rather, the teachers paid their monthly premium in exchange for a *service* that the hospital would provide when and if a teacher needed it. The service had already been paid for—in advance; it was "prepaid."

In 1932 (the worst year of the Great Depression) the three major private, nonprofit hospitals in the Sacramento, California, area agreed on a joint hospitalization plan, which they then offered to local employee groups. Not only did this community-wide plan make its sponsoring hospitals happy by paying some of their patients' bills, it also avoided the inter-hospital competition that was inevitable whenever a single hospital plan, like the one in Dallas, offered itself to employee groups. The Sacramento plan gave the patients a choice of any of the three local hospitals (and, thus, their choice of doctors as well). Community-wide, nonprofit "hospital service plans" spread rapidly throughout the country, and with the backing of state hospital associations they soon consolidated into state-wide or metropolitan area–wide plans. In 1934 one of them adopted a logo with a blue cross on it, and soon that's what they were calling themselves.

The new "Blue Cross" hospital service plans offered something they called *service benefits*. Unlike indemnity insurance, which paid (indemnified) patients a certain amount after they presented a bill, *service benefit plans* paid hospitals directly. This is why the Blue Cross plans did not originally consider themselves "insurance companies" at all. Although most of them also eventually provided traditional insurance products, their hospital "service benefit" tradition remained—and still remains—strong. Listen to the television commercials for Blue Cross or look at its ads in the newspaper. You will never hear or read the word "insurance." Again, this is because the Blue Cross plans were not set up to compensate the insured person for a loss. Patients didn't submit claims; hospitals did. This difference was a very important one to Blue Cross. And it was an equally important issue for the organized medical profession, since the doctors feared the control that being paid directly by an "insurance" plan would bring or that it implied might come.

The commercial insurance companies watched the beginnings of Blue Cross with skepticism. They had been reluctant to offer health insurance themselves, because they saw so many problems with it—the high expenses of paying commissions to a force of sales agents, the expense of collecting the premium each month, the issue of how to control abuse (the question, again, of exactly what is the "indemnity" in health care) and, especially, the fear that those who purchased health insurance would do so because they were already sick or likely to become sick; the insurance companies called this problem "adverse selection." Yet, contrary to the insurance industry's expectation that Blue Cross would fail, it grew rapidly—so rapidly that by the late 1930s the commercial carriers were sufficiently impressed that they, too, began offering hospitalization coverage to employee groups. (Blue Cross had by then demonstrated that *group* coverage could largely eliminate the "adverse selection" problem.) Unlike the Blue Cross policies, which paid service benefits, the hospitalization coverage offered by the commercial carriers was in the form of traditional indemnity insurance.

During all this time the American Medical Association watched the new Blue Cross plans warily. It warned them to stick to covering hospital expenses and not try branching out to include medical services. The AMA objected to doctors being paid by a plan—any plan. It would however be acceptable, the AMA said, for cash benefits to be paid directly to the individual member (the insured patient), since that would not disturb "the relations of patients and physicians." But doctors were not to be involved. In other words, indemnity plans, but not service benefit plans, could cover medical services. Soon the commercial insurance companies began listing surgeons' fees as a benefit covered by their group policies.

Later, the AMA changed its position and said that service benefits might be acceptable, but only if medical societies controlled the plans. So medical society–sponsored plans, which covered surgical and medical services provided during hospitalization, were established during the 1940s. They called themselves "Blue Shield" plans. Blue Cross helped many of them get started and even provided their administrative staffs. There was a good reason why Blue Cross was so willing to lend assistance. By offering Blue Cross *and* Blue Shield benefits in a single package, Blue Cross could maintain the competitive edge that its older "service benefit" plans enjoyed over the younger, but rapidly growing commercial "indemnity" plans.

The Third Way: Direct Service Plans (1900–1970)

Direct service plans are actually the oldest of the three kinds of private health "insurance" in the United States. They started well before the others but grew more slowly—until the 1970s, when their growth accelerated.

With direct service plans moral hazard was never an issue, because these plans were not insurance. In contrast with traditional indemnity insurance, which compensated the insured for a loss, and service benefit plans, which paid "costs" incurred by hospitals or fees to physicians, direct service plans actually saw to it that the needed service was delivered to the patient. They paid their benefits not in the form of money—to either patient or provider—but rather in the form of direct services. The reason they could do this is that they employed, or contracted with, or owned all of the service resources—physicians, hospitals, laboratories, and so on—their enrolled members were likely to need. Nor were the huge cash reserves required of indemnity insurance companies and Blue Cross necessary for direct service plans, since their benefits were not paid as cash disbursements, but rather as entitled services from hospitals and doctors whose service delivery capacity had been "reserved" for the plan's members. So in a sense, these plans weren't selling insurance at all, but "assurance." Of course, the members faced a restriction: under the plan they could only use the plan's own doctors and hospitals. And the medical work was naturally monitored closely by the plan. For these two reasons, the organized medical profession seldom held a favorable opinion of direct service plans.

The mutual benefit societies in Europe and their counterparts in certain American cities around the turn of the 20th century were direct service plans. (The members, collectively, contracted with a doctor who then served them when they fell ill.) The major, early direct service plans in America, however, were almost all in nonurban locations. Why? Because this is where extractive industries are commonly found; they tend to be intensive operations requiring large numbers of workers, and they are dangerous industries. Since there weren't enough doctors in these locations, and since the employers realized that an unhealthy workforce could not be a productive workforce, the companies who located in these out-of-the-way places had to find a way of attracting physicians. They did this by, in effect, guaranteeing the doctors a clientele consisting of the workers, who would pay the doctors in advance through what was called a "check-off" system (a regular amount deducted from the workers' paychecks). Sometimes the company contracted with the doctors; sometimes it employed them. From the late 19th century until well after World War II, direct service plans were operated by mines, railroads, lumber companies, fisheries, and the large construction firms that built the dams and aqueducts in the far West.

Enrollment in virtually all of the early industrial direct service plans was limited to the sponsoring company's own employees and sometimes their dependents—until 1929. In that year (the same year the Baylor University Hospital started its prepaid hospitalization plan) two new direct service plans started; both were organized around group medical practice, but they provided hospital service as well; and both plans opened themselves to the general public. One was operated by the Ross-Loos Medical Group of Los Angeles; the other was a Farmer's Union–sponsored cooperative hospital in Elk City, Oklahoma. In spite of harassment by organized medicine—the physicians in both groups were expelled from their county medical societies, resulting in, among other things, an inability to purchase malpractice insurance—both succeeded.

Although a few other direct service plans opened during the 1930s, "prepaid group practice," as these plans later called themselves, grew hardly at all until just after World War II, when the Kaiser-Permanente Health Plans on the West Coast, the Group Health Cooperative of Puget Sound in Seattle, and the Health Insurance Plan (HIP) of Greater New York began enrolling the general public—especially members of labor unions—in direct competition with the Blues and the commercial carriers.[13]

One problem that prepaid group practice plans faced wherever they opened was opposition from the local medical profession. Another problem was the huge capital expenditures that were required to start a new multispecialty medical group from scratch. On the other hand, the prepaid group practice plans held a major advantage over the commercial indemnity plans and the Blues: they could deliver care of higher quality at lower cost. Research reports documenting this advantage began appearing in the 1950s; but it wasn't until the early 1970s, after the federal government discovered a medical care cost crisis, that their cost advantage translated into a national policy favoring direct service plans. The Nixon administration began promoting direct service plans as a way of curbing the rapidly escalating costs of medical care. It also gave them a new name: *health maintenance organizations* or *HMOs*.

Social Insurance and President Roosevelt (1935–1938)

In 1934 President Franklin D. Roosevelt appointed a cabinet committee, chaired by Labor secretary Francis Perkins, to study social insurance and bring back recommendations for legislation. The committee was to consider three categories of social insurance: unemployment insurance, old-age pensions, and health insurance. Although the health insurance sub-committee recommended that a compulsory, state-by-state program be part of the Social Security Bill, President Roosevelt excluded it from the final version. His reason had to do with the AMA's opposition. What the doctors had learned of the subcommittee's work raised their antibody titer to the point that the AMA's trustees called an unprecedented emergency session of the House of Delegates. And so when the president considered the probable strength of the doctors' opposition, he guessed that the health insurance provision could well be an albatross that would sink the entire bill.

Yet, while the Social Security Act of 1935 didn't include health insurance, it did other things in health care, like reviving (and expanding) the maternal and child care provisions of the old Sheppard-Towner Act. It also gave federal grants to the states that put public health departments on a sound basis; and it established the Crippled Children's Program.

The main feature of the Social Security Act was, of course, its old-age pensions provision—the provision that Americans first think of when they hear the words "social security." In this respect the United States broke with the pattern that the European nations had generally followed. Social security enactment had usually begun in these other countries with *protection against industrial accidents* (workmen's compensation); and here America followed suit. Next came *protection against the costs of illness* (sickness insurance in the form of cash payments for time lost from work), followed by *protection against the costs of medical and hospital bills* (health insurance). But only after these social insurance programs were in place did most European nations enact *protection against the inability to earn a living in old age* (old-age pensions) and *protection against loss of income due to losing one's job* (unemployment insurance).

In the United States health insurance was to have been next, after workmen's compensation. Even after the AALL campaign failed, health insurance remained the next item of business on the social reformers' agenda. But then came the depression, which not only put millions of people out of work, it also stirred up a political movement for old-age pensions. The consequence was that in America unemployment insurance came second—the states began enacting it in 1932—and following close behind came the old-age pensions in the Social Security Act of 1935.

Once President Roosevelt dropped health insurance from his Social Security Bill, he never again made it part of his legislative program. In fact, he backed away from it again, in 1938, after his National Health Conference had recommended essentially the same proposal that the health insurance subcommittee of the Perkins Committee had advanced back in 1934. FDR presumably hoped to push health insurance in the wake of that 1938 conference, but war broke out the next year, the president's priorities changed, and social insurance for health care once more dropped off the American agenda.

Social Insurance: The Truman Program (1945–1950)

Social insurance for health care reappeared after the war, when President Truman gave his support to the second Wagner-Murray-Dingell Bill, which proposed national health insurance under Social Security (what we now call a "single-payer" program). When someone asked how he'd pay for it, Truman replied that he thought the American people could afford to spend more than the 4% of gross domestic product (GDP) that the nation was then spending on health care. In 1945 escalation of health care costs was not seen as a problem.[14]

The three Wagner-Murray-Dingell bills and the Truman plan all advanced essentially the same program—compulsory national health insurance under Social Security. Three decades earlier, at the time of the AALL's state-by-state plan, when the main "risk of work" was the likelihood of the breadwinner's missing a paycheck because of illness, it was natural that workers' health insurance would have been linked to their employment. By 1934—when state-by-state health insurance next appeared on the national agenda—it had become less natural to link it to employment (since by this time the risk of missed work had been joined by a second problem; the burden of an expense, borne by a patient—an expense that relates only marginally to the patient's employment). It wasn't until the 1940s that a major health insurance proposal clearly *unlinked* people's health coverage from their employment. Wagner-Murray-Dingell proposed a national compulsory program linked to Social Security; the premium would have been collected and paid just as the old-age pension premium was: through the employer (or by the self-employed worker); but seeking the needed care—including the question of "choice" of physician or hospital—would have had no more to do with one's employment than would the choice of bank into which a pensioner deposited her or his monthly social security check.

When President Truman made national health insurance an issue in the 1948 presidential campaign, the AMA was concerned, but not overly so; its antibody titer rose only slightly. The doctors believed, along with nearly everyone else, that the president would be defeated in the fall election by the Republican candidate, New York Governor Thomas Dewey, and that would be that. But Truman was elected, and so was, again, a Democratic Congress.

When the election results became known, organized medicine panicked and launched a massive national publicity campaign that capitalized on the anticommunist hysteria that was then permeating the country. The AMA called the Truman plan *socialized medicine*, unashamedly equated it with communism, and raised the specter of enslaved doctors operating on unwilling patients. That kind of propaganda was effective in 1949.[15]

Yet, even without the AMA's opposition, the Truman plan for a national health insurance program stood little chance politically. The forces aligned against it were simply too powerful. Big business and the Republican Party both opposed national health insurance, and so did most of the southern congressional Democrats, who not only chaired the key committees but also, with the Republicans, made up a conservative majority in both houses of Congress.

The reason the Truman health insurance plan failed, however, may have had less to do with the strength of the political opposition than with the rapid growth of private insurance. In 1940, only about 7% of Americans had any health insurance coverage of any kind. By 1975, only 35 years later, nearly everyone was covered. But the most rapid period of growth came between the end of the war and 1950—during the Truman years. So it is understandable that in 1949 the most effective argument against the Truman plan was that social health insurance wasn't needed, because soon everyone would be covered by voluntary, private health insurance.

The Effect of World War II on Private Health Insurance
(1939–1945)

At least four factors were responsible for this prodigious growth in private health insurance coverage just after the war. The first was a policy decision that came just *before* the war. The second had to do with a series of government decisions about taxes, wages, and prices made *during* the war. The third was the experience of the American servicemen who fought the war. And the fourth was a change in strategy on the part of organized labor in the immediate postwar years. These four factors, taken together, not only explain much of the growth in private insurance during the late 1940s and throughout the 1950s; they also go a long way toward explaining how it is that Americans came to have the health system they do today.

Back in 1939 the Internal Revenue Service made a ruling that allowed an employer to deduct the cost of paying employee fringe benefits from the employer's taxable income. The IRS said that fringe benefits were a business expense for the company and not a portion of the employees' incomes (which would have made them subject to personal income tax). Nor, the IRS ruled, would the value of these fringe benefits be considered part of the base for computing the Social Security tax.

This was a momentous decision, although at the time it didn't seem that important, since in 1939 few employers were providing worker benefits of any kind. Unions weren't pressing for benefits then either; they had long considered fringe benefits to be an employer's way of ducking its real responsibility of paying the workers a fair wage. Further, in 1939 most business employers were still feeling the effects of the Great Depression and were not eager to pay for employee benefits. The main effect of the IRS decision would come later.

Following America's entry into World War II on December 7, 1941, millions of young Americans were in uniform. But the war was also responsible for another "army" of civilian workers, who joined in a massive migration, mostly from rural to urban areas, to take jobs in the defense industry. People went to Los Angeles, Portland, Mobile, Baltimore, Norfolk, Oakland, Detroit, Worcester, Pittsburgh, Peoria, Seattle, Ft. Worth, Wichita, Denver, and hundreds of other cities and smaller places where defense industries were expanding. Some of these towns saw their populations double within a few months. The depression was over; instead of a job shortage the nation faced a labor shortage.

At this point, the government took a notable action. It came from the National War Labor Board, one of two new wartime inflation watchdog agencies; the other one was the Office of Price Administration. One agency watched wages; the other watched prices. The purpose of both agencies was to curb inflation. It is critically important during wartime to guard against inflation, because all of the major factors that bring it about are present. Demand is high because of the war; supply (of both goods and services to the home front) is low because of the war; and labor is in short supply—also because of the war. The War Labor Board also had another job—preventing strikes; work stoppages would obviously hamper the war production effort. The most direct way of curbing inflation is limiting both wage increases and price increases. The best way to prevent strikes—the best democratic way, because in a free society government can't command people to work—was to mollify the unions. Satisfying unions while at the same time prohibiting wage increases is not easy.

In the summer of 1942, the War Labor Board announced a rule. It said that wages could rise by no more than 15% above the levels that were in effect in January of 1941, and that once a company's employees had received that 15% raise, their wages would be essentially frozen for the duration of the war. This meant that at a time when the national unemployment rate was only 2%, when keeping workers was a major problem for employers, they could no longer use the carrot of higher wages to recruit workers. The companies weren't happy with the War Labor Board's rule; neither were the unions satisfied with the 15% limit, especially when they saw how much the companies were likely to earn (despite the excess profits tax) from their cost-plus government contracts.

In response to the complaints, the War Labor Board handed down a further decision later in 1942. The board reiterated its earlier ruling that any wage increases beyond the 15% limit were out of the question. But it then added a new proviso: some additional benefits or "fringe adjustments" (adjustments like vacations and day care and health insurance) would not be considered inflationary and would therefore not count as wage increases against the 15% limit. With this decision the floodgates opened. Unions and management both sought wage increases under the guise of "fringe adjustments." By the end of the war, the number of American workers covered by health insurance had tripled.

Private Insurance after the War (1945–1955)

Meanwhile, 15 million soldiers and at least a couple of million dependents had been receiving their medical care from the military. For the vast majority, military medicine was better than anything they had ever experienced before. It was accessible, of high quality, and best of all, it didn't cost them anything. Military medicine during the war was well organized and highly effective. If a soldier was wounded in combat and a corpsman could get to him, the wounded soldier had a 93% chance of surviving. And at the end of the war, before a serviceman was mustered out he was examined thoroughly and he received whatever treatment he needed from qualified specialists in efficient hospitals.

In addition to providing America's soldiers and sailors with whatever medical care they required, military medicine raised their expectations. When the war was over and many of them became baby boomer parents, these veterans wanted the same access to medical care for their families that they had enjoyed themselves while in the service. So the postwar expectations of World War II veterans constituted yet another force pushing the growth of private health insurance.

But perhaps the most important postwar boost for employment-based health insurance came from the growth and consequent strength of organized labor. With the war had come economic prosperity; employers stopped worrying about fighting unions: they had a more important concern—how to keep up production. Anyhow, cost-plus government contracts and government wage and price controls had largely relieved the pressure of worker demands for higher wages. Meanwhile, the unions grew, adding nearly 6 million new workers to their membership rolls during the war (between 1940 and 1945).

When the war ended the economy continued to boom. Some prominent economists predicted that peace would bring recession. It didn't. One precept of economics is that full employment and rising wages leads to more consumption of goods and services. During the war there was certainly full employment, and wages rose by at least the allowed 15%. But contrary to the rule, these conditions had not led to a great increase in domestic purchasing—for a simple reason: there was little that workers could buy. Car manufacturers had been making tanks and planes; and staples like rubber, aluminum, and steel were all directed to the war effort; gasoline and food were rationed. And, of course, a sizable portion of the population was in uniform and living off GI (government issue). When the war ended, the pent-up demand for consumer goods was tremendous. Further, when the price and wage controls ended—the same day the war ended—inflation followed. Naturally, the labor unions wanted to make sure that workers' wages would keep up with the rising prices. For the most part, their wages did keep up, to the point that many workers were earning enough to pay income tax for the first time in their lives. The workers didn't achieve this gain, however, without a great deal of militant, industrial action. The peak year for strikes in American history was 1946.

The reason why labor began to push for *private* social security had to do with the vagaries of politics. American workers had favored *public* (government) social security from the time of the Social Security Act in 1935. And labor unions were major participants in the campaign to expand it to include health insurance; organized labor had backed the first Wagner-Murray-Dingell bill, introduced in 1943. When the second Wagner-Murray-Dingell bill came along in 1945 and 1946—essentially a reintroduction of the first one—most union leaders thought it would pass, just as the British labor unions at this same time were expecting the British National Health Service to be enacted (it was, in 1948). But the United States followed a different postwar political course than the British.

In the fall of 1946, the Republicans prevailed in the midterm elections and took control of both houses of Congress for the first time since 1931. Part of the reason was the general dissatisfaction felt by the American people with the unusual and unseemly labor agitation of that year. In 1947, the Republican Congress passed the antiunion Taft-Hartley Bill over President Truman's veto.

At this point the labor unions had to reassess their strategy. They had lost the election and the battle over Taft-Hartley; and it now looked like national health insurance wasn't going to arrive any time soon. Both the president of the CIO (Congress of Industrial Organizations) and the president of the AFL (American Federation of Labor) agreed that labor, in the words of the AFL president, "would have no other recourse than to demand private welfare plans from private employers." The unions changed course: they began to bargain not just for wages, but now also for welfare benefits—retirement pensions, disability benefits, health insurance.

The employers didn't care for this change in strategy. They had come to accept the notion that unions would represent the workers in bargaining over wages.[16] But bargaining over benefits was different; in their view it overstepped an important boundary between management and labor. American corporations were accustomed to providing benefits as a way of winning and keeping worker loyalty; benefits were a management prerogative, and not something to be put on the bargaining table.

The employers argued that the Wagner Act (the original National Labor Relations Act of 1935) had said only that workers could bargain for "wages, hours, and other terms or conditions of employment." The act said nothing about bargaining over employee benefits. And benefits, the employers argued, were not and never had been "conditions of employment." The unions disagreed.

The dispute was settled after Inland Steel refused to bargain with the United Steelworkers of America over some changes the union wanted to make in the pension plan. The union called a strike and appealed to the National Labor Relations Board (NLRB), which handed down its ruling in

1948. A pension, it said, could indeed be considered a "term or condition of employment." The result was that during the decade of the 1950s, unions proceeded to bargain for and managed to gain more liberal health insurance benefits for their members than they had enjoyed previously. This then meant that many nonunion employers had to match what the unions had won.

The outcome of the decisions made by the federal government (by the IRS, the War Labor Board, and the NLRB) before, during and just after World War II; the raised expectations of returning servicemen; and the push of organized labor to bargain for benefits after the unions failed to win the political victory they most wanted was this: instead of the *social* health insurance systems that other high-income, industrialized nations were building or already had in place by the 1940s and 1950s, the United States developed an alternative, employer-based system of *private* health insurance.

The Fragmentation of the Risk Pool (1948–1958)

At the time of the NLRB's 1948 decision in the Steelworkers–Inland Steel dispute, the older, nonprofit Blue Cross plans were dominating the newer commercial health insurance plans. Yet, the commercial companies were successful in capturing a large share of the new employment-based health insurance market. Much of the reason for their success had to do with the important concepts of *community rating* and *experience rating*. These are two basic methods that insurance carriers use to set the amount of the premium. It is important to understand the difference between them and the consequences of adopting either one.

Under *community rating*, the entire population of an area is charged the same rate, regardless of their risk as individuals of becoming ill. People who are more likely to become sick are subsidized by those who are more likely to remain healthy, since the sickness-prone people don't pay a higher premium than the others, even though they will probably use doctors and hospitals more.

Under *experience rating* the entire population is not even considered as a group; instead it is divided into subgroups (usually corresponding to the employees of a company). Each subgroup is then charged its own rate, based upon how likely the members are to become ill. In this way, insurance companies are able to charge lower rates to the subgroups that are made up of mostly healthy people and charge higher rates to subgroups that contain a greater proportion of less healthy people—who are sick or have been sick in the past, or who are members of known high risk populations such as the poor and the elderly. An insurance company's actuaries can predict how much medical care each subgroup is likely to use, and the company can thereby quote a premium that reflects this actuarial risk.

The essential difference between community rating and experience rating is, however, not so much in how the premium is set but in how the risk is pooled. If either rating method were to be applied to the entire population, the effects would be dramatic.

One way to understand this is to consider how things would be under what we might call the socialist ideal, or Christian ideal (depending on your view—both groups, plus several others, claim original authorship of the idea but none has yet demonstrated its full implementation). Those most able to give would *give* the most, and those with the greatest need would *take* the most. Thus, the poorest and sickest would give little but take a lot, while the most wealthy and healthy would give a lot but take little.

By contrast, one's *ability to give* is not a consideration under either community rating or experience rating. Community rating demands that everyone pay the same; but those who are least healthy may take more, while the healthiest would naturally take less. Under experience rating, the healthiest people would again take the least, but they could also expect to pay less; on the other hand, the least healthy would take the most, but in return they would have to pay the most.

Social health insurance programs like Germany's and Great Britain's had always charged the same premium for health insurance to old people and young people, and to coal miners, dressmakers, railway ticket clerks, and steeplejacks. So had the Blue Cross plans, which began as a community-wide hospital service associations charging everyone the same "community rate." Both national health insurance plans and Blue Cross were unwilling to isolate workers according to risk. But the commercial insurance companies *were* willing to isolate workers, and everyone else, by risk. To them, experience rating for health insurance seemed no different than what they had always done in their life insurance business, charging more to cover old people who are near the end of life, or in their casualty insurance business, quoting a lower fire insurance premium for the house that is located next door to the engine house.

Active workers are on average young and healthy and therefore likely to use less medical care (unless they are in high-risk occupations like coal mining). So by isolating the illness experience of groups of active workers from that of the rest of the community, the commercial insurance company could quote a premium that would be as low as possible while still allowing the company to make a predictable profit from each group.

When employers discovered that their employees' collective health risk was below that of the community as a whole, they wanted rates that reflected this more favorable experience. Unions wanted the same thing. Soon the commercial companies began to overtake the Blues in writing group health insurance. It wasn't long before the Blues realized that if they expected to compete for the large employment-based group insurance market, they would have to adopt experience rating themselves.

Here is a principle: the more fragmented the risk pool becomes, the more difficult it is for those left in the *common pool* to find affordable health insurance. Throughout the 1950s, as unions and employers purchased health plans that used experience rating, they left behind a community risk pool that included a greater proportion of the poor and marginally employed, the sick and disabled, and, especially, the elderly. When the most attractive members of society from a risk standpoint are covered under an experience rating system, their premium will, naturally, be less. At the same time the average risk of illness among the "community" left behind rises. Since the experience of the healthiest group is no longer being factored into the community rate, the premium for those who remain in the community pool—the residue—also rises until, finally, they find themselves priced out of the private health insurance market.

The Road to Medicare (1958–1965)

That is what happened to the elderly during the 1950s. When they retired, most of them lost their employer-provided health insurance. And all of this was happening at a time when the cost of an acute-care hospital admission was rising rapidly.

In 1958 a Rhode Island Congressman named Aime Forand introduced a bill to insure the elderly for hospitalization under Social Security. President Eisenhower opposed it. However, presidential candidate Kennedy supported the idea. In fact, social health insurance for the elderly became a minor issue in the 1960 presidential campaign between Senator Kennedy and Vice President Nixon. Kennedy favored the King-Anderson Bill (the successor to the Forand Bill), while Nixon supported another plan

(Kerr-Mills) by which the federal government would help the states provide additional public assistance (welfare) to the elderly poor to help them pay hospital bills.

After Kennedy became president he tried to get King-Anderson passed, but there wasn't enough congressional support. The AMA vigorously opposed it, and at that time the AMA, with about 175,000 doctor members, had the second largest (measured by expenditures) political lobbying organization in Washington, second only to the AFL-CIO, which in the early 1960s represented nearly 16 *million* labor union members.[17]

After the 1964 election the necessary congressional support was there, and President Johnson signed the *Medicare* bill into law the following year.[18] To the original Forand Bill and the successor King-Anderson Bill, which covered only hospital service, Medicare added a voluntary but generously subsidized (from general tax revenue) "Part B," which paid for the services of physicians.[19] The new law also included a public assistance program for the poor called *Medicaid*—operated by the states but jointly funded by federal and state governments.

President Johnson's forceful personality and political skills were critically important to the passage of Medicare. But it was a popular grassroots campaign by the nation's elderly, backed by organized labor and other organizations—the same coalition that had supported President Truman's program 17 years earlier—that really forced the issue. On the other side, the bill's most vigorous opponent was the AMA. It lobbied, advertised, and even sent doctors' wives anti-Medicare phonograph records and tapes to play for their neighbors.[20] But this time, organized medicine's antibody titer against social insurance wasn't high enough to defeat it. Before long, the doctors liked Medicare well enough; it sent their incomes soaring.

After Medicare

After Medicare was implemented in July of 1966 it appeared to many that the United States had in place a satisfactory system of medical care financing, consisting of voluntary private health insurance for most employed people, welfare medical care for the poor and marginally employed, and social health insurance for the elderly.

But soon a problem arose that has preoccupied American health policy makers to the end of the 20th century and beyond: escalating medical care costs and how to contain them. Controlling costs was one of two main issues of medical care payment that have prevailed throughout the post-

Medicare period. The other issue, which arose long before Medicare, was how to provide financial access to care for more Americans. Almost always the latter question has prompted renewed proposals for some form of social insurance. The access-social insurance issue has appeared on the national policy agenda through 18 presidential terms (covered by 12 presidents). Several of those presidents announced their intentions to expand social insurance for health care. Some—Roosevelt, Nixon, Ford and Carter—failed to make the strong effort it would have required. Others, like Eisenhower, Reagan and both presidents Bush, either denied that a problem existed or opposed social insurance as a solution. Presidents Truman, Kennedy, and Clinton tried but failed; only one president—Lyndon Johnson—succeeded.

Starting with Nixon, every president has also faced the problem of runaway costs. By 1969 the apparent uncontrollability of medical care costs had become the health policy issue that drowned out all others. That was when President Nixon declared that American health care was in a state of crisis, and opinion polls showed that 75% of Americans agreed. By 1969, total annual health care expenditures were 7.3% of GDP. (Remember that President Truman had said in 1945 that the nation could afford to spend more than the 4% of GDP then being spent on health care.)

Some presidents (and other politicians and experts) have placed their faith in "competition" or "markets" for controlling medical care costs; others have favored mild regulation. Both strategies were tried, with the result that health care expenditures rose over the past two decades to somewhere between 13 and 14% of GDP—proving that Nixon's characterization of a "crisis" back in 1969 was correct.

Since then, and in response to that "crisis," America's patterns of payment for medical care have become far more complex, to the point that one can fairly characterize these multifarious payment mechanisms as constituting another kind of crisis: we now must contend with an enormous and confusing variety of "managed care products"—all of them descendents, hybrids, or other relatives of the three original varieties of private insurance. Government programs (Medicare and Medicaid) offer these products to eligible citizens in the name of "choice"; employers choose them for their employees in the name of controlling business expenses.

Meanwhile, as health care costs continue to rise relative to the economy as a whole, the number of Americans who must live unprotected by some form of health coverage also grows. And those who *do* have employment-based health insurance see their "choice" narrow and their protective cover shrink—by an increase in the out-of-pocket deductible and co-insurance they must pay, or through a diminished scope of benefits from their employer-sponsored plan.

By any measure, medical care costs far more today than it used to. There are many reasons, but the first is that the service itself is so much more complex. Yet, it doesn't follow that payment need be equally complex; it isn't so in other nations, where medical professionals use the same technology. America could adopt any number of national models—from Canada's to Denmark's to Japan's—and thereby cover all its citizens and achieve greater simplicity of the system.

With respect to universal coverage, however, the United States has for nearly a century been the holdout among industrialized nations. We may yet see universal coverage; but if we do, if history is a guide, we should not expect to see any great change in how the system is organized. For except following full-scale political revolution or major political shifts in the wake of war, no nation has ever enacted a program of social insurance for health care that did not build on whatever incomplete private system was already in place. This was true of the programs enacted by Bismarck and Lloyd George, as we have seen. It was true in this country, as well, in the case of Medicare, which built on the Blue Cross system of hospital payment and the private indemnity insurance system of paying physicians.

The American private system of medical care payment has changed dramatically since the enactment of Medicare. It is now dominated by an aggressive, highly competitive private sector that responds hardly at all, except defensively, to political pressure and acts forcefully to edify its corporate organizational culture. Whether or not this is a desirable direction is a matter of opinion, of where one sits. We must expect, however, that any future program of universal—or merely expanded—coverage will build on our present corporate-style private system or whatever it evolves into.

Notes

1 Sir William Beveridge, author of the wartime Beveridge Report (1942), articulated the conceptual and political foundations of the British National Health Service (enacted six years later). Sigerist was placing this contemporary development in historical context. Henry E. Sigerist, "From Bismarck to Beveridge: Developments and Trends in Social Security Legislation," *Bulletin of the History of Medicine* 8 (April 1943): 365–388.

2 This idea also comes from Sigerist the historian, who was also a social activist and a serious student of contemporary medical care, and who taught his courses in social policy and medical care organization from a historical perspective.

3 I say "his wife" because "once upon a time" that gender relationship would have been true 99 times out of 100.

4 A few years ago hospitals accounted for half of all medical care costs in the United States. Certain complex diagnostic and treatment modalities that were once rendered only in the hospital are now routinely performed on an outpatient (ambulatory care) basis. This change explains the relative decrease.

5 There are two excellent book-length accounts of the AALL episode. The first, by Ronald Numbers, deals with the responses of the medical profession (*Almost Persuaded: American Physicians and Compulsory Health Insurance, 1912–1920* [Baltimore: Johns Hopkins University Press, 1978]). The second, by Beatrix Hoffman, relates the political history of the campaign in the State of New York (*The Wages of Sickness: The Politics of Health Insurance in Progressive America* [Chapel Hill: University of North Carolina Press, 2001]).

6 John J. A. O'Reilly to the Medical Society of the County of Kings, New York, October 21, 1919. Quoted (capital letters included) in Ronald L. Numbers, *Almost Persuaded: American Physicians and Compulsory Health Insurance, 1912–1920*, p. 93.

7 Minutes of the House of Delegates, *Journal of the American Medical Association* 74 (May 8, 1920): 1319.

8 The mutual benefit society never became established in America the way it did in Europe. It did enjoy some popularity among groups of immigrants attempting to replicate the self-help institutions they knew from the old country.

9 By 1920 many American industrial firms were providing on-the-job medical care. The more expansive company-sponsored programs were part of an important but temporary chapter in the history of American labor-management relations that the unions called "industrial paternalism" and that historians now refer to as "welfare capitalism." Many welfare capitalism programs provided modest public health services. Only two—the Tennessee Coal and Iron Company, operating around Birmingham, Alabama, and the Endicott Johnson Corporation, around Binghamton, New York—sponsored complete medical care programs, as good as existed anywhere. A general history of welfare capitalism is Stuart D. Brandes, *American Welfare Capitalism, 1880–1940* (Chicago: University of Chicago Press, 1976).

10 At the end of the 1920s only two specialties—ophthalmology and otolaryngology—had formal specialty boards. However, many physicians practiced as specialists in virtually all of the branches of medicine that over the next 10 years would form boards and be recognized as formal specialties.

11 From the "Preface on Doctors" to *The Doctor's Dilemma*.

12 Commercial fire insurance first found a market following the Great Fire of London (1666). Life insurance companies emerged in the late 1840s. A few of them also sold health insurance (sickness insurance) beginning around the turn of the 20th century, but only to their life policyholders; they saw their sickness insurance offerings as a marketing ploy for their life insurance products, not as an independent line from which they expected to profit.

13 Kaiser had existed during the war as an industrial plan for Kaiser shipyard and steel workers. The forerunner of Group Health in Seattle had also operated as a wartime industrial plan. HIP, however, was organized *de novo* during the 1940s, largely under the personal

sponsorship of New York mayor Fiorello La Guardia. It was financed by loans from several foundations, principally Rockefeller.

14 The Gross Domestic Product or GDP is the value of all goods and services produced in the nation. The rate at which the GDP grows or recedes is a measure of the nation's economic health: in good times it expands; during recessions it lags. But since the entire GDP can never be larger than 100%, knowing the portion of it that a particular sector of the economy occupies tells how much is left for everything else people need or want—individually or collectively. For example, if we had to spend 30% of our total national wealth on housing, we would have only 70% left for national defense, college tuition, shoes, interest on the national debt, food, repairing roads and bridges, church offerings, movie tickets, medical care, and everything else we must have or would like to have.

15 Several events of 1949 underlined the gravity of the cold war: The Berlin Blockade, the communist takeover of China, and the explosion by the Soviet Union of a first atomic bomb. The following year saw the beginning of both the Korean War and Senator Joseph McCarthy's communist witch hunt.

16 The National Relations Act of 1935 required employers to bargain in good faith with a union that their employees had elected to represent them.

17 The AFL-CIO was formed in 1955 when the two rival labor organizations merged.

18 Lyndon Johnson's landslide defeat of Republican candidate Barry Goldwater (Johnson lost only Goldwater's home state of Arizona and five states in the deep South) swept into office a large number of congressional Democrats. In the 89th Congress Democrats outnumbered Republicans by more than two to one in both the House and Senate. The conservative coalition that for so long had long bottled up social welfare initiatives, including the Truman plan, was broken.

19 Although those who elect to participate in Part B must pay a monthly premium (deducted from the Social Security check), the federal subsidy is so generous that almost everyone does elect it. Further, since most private retirement medical care plans and "medigap" politics are linked to Part B, it is effectively mandatory for millions of Medicare participants.

20 The public relations consultants who came up with this campaign named it "Operation Coffee Cup."

The Sad History of Health Care Cost Containment as Told in One Chart

Drew E. Altman and Larry Levitt

The problem of rising health care costs is reemerging as a national issue. Unfortunately, costs are rising as the economy sputters, the federal surplus dwindles, and the nation is focused on the war against terrorism and its ripple effects here at home. It will now be much harder to make much progress on big-ticket health problems such as expanding health coverage for the uninsured and providing drug coverage for seniors.

Many lament what they believe has been a failure of managed care to control health costs. That criticism may or may not be accurate or fair, but it is almost certainly short-sighted. What the analysis of private health spending reported in figure 1 shows is that no approach our nation has tried, over the past 35 years, to control health costs has had a lasting impact. When Medicare and Medicaid passed in the mid-1960s, the new public programs took some of the burden of health spending off of the private sector, but only temporarily. By the late 1960s the rate of increase in private health spending per capita shot up. In the early 1970s wage and price controls had a dramatic impact on health care costs. But again, the impact was short-lived, and the rate of increase in private health spending rose dramatically after a few years. When President Jimmy Carter threatened tough cost containment regulation in the late 1970s, the health care industry organized what it called the "Voluntary Effort." The rate of increase in per capita private-sector health spending fell rapidly but then bounced back within a few years. Managed care and the threat of the Clinton health care reform plan appeared to have had a dramatic impact on the rate of increase in private health spending in the mid-1990s, but by

Drew E. Altman and Larry Levitt, "The Sad History of Health Care Cost Containment as Told in One Chart," from *Health Affairs*, Web Exclusive, 23 January 2002, 83–84. © 2002 by Project HOPE—The People-to-People Health Foundation, Inc.

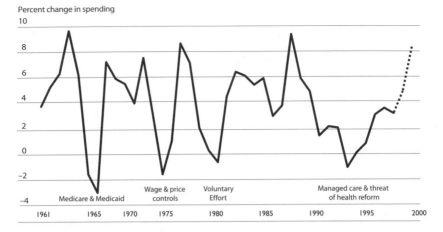

Percent change in spending

Figure 1. Annual Change in Private Health Spending per Capita (Adjusted for Inflation), 1961–2001. Sources: Henry J. Kaiser Family Foundation analysis. Private health expenditures per capita, 1960–1999, are from the Centers for Medicare and Medicaid Services (CMS). Change in private spending per capita, 2000–2001, is estimated based on average premium increases for employer-sponsored coverage from the Kaiser/HRET Survey of Employer-Sponsored Health Benefits. Notes: Real change in spending is calculated using the Consumer Price Index (CPI-U) on all items, average annual change for 1961–2000 and July-to-July change for 2001. This analysis was inspired by an analysis done by Jeff Merrill and Richard Wassermann more than fifteen years ago. See J. C. Merrill and R. J. Wassermann, "Growth in National Expenditures: Additional Analyses," *Health Affairs* (Winter 1985): 91–98.

the late 1990s it was on the rise again, reaching double-digit rates of increase by 2001.

In sum, neither regulation, voluntary action by the health care industry, nor managed care and market competition have had a lasting impact on our nation's health care costs. Some might argue that we were not serious or comprehensive enough about any one of these approaches for them to have had a lasting impact. On the other hand, it could be argued that the point is academic; we were as serious as public and political support for any one approach would allow.

Some believe that we will not get a handle on health care costs as a nation until we are ready to make tough decisions about rationing medical care. An equally plausible scenario is that the apparent failure of all approaches reflects the American people's uncontainable desire for the latest and best health care, and that what we will do in the future is try small things that will work at the margin, complain a lot, but ultimately pay the bill. Whichever view is right, the historical data, while certainly open to different interpretations, show that managed care is not alone in its failure to solve the health care cost problem. Indeed, history suggests that it may be folly to expect that there are any easy or magic answers to this problem. When it comes to controlling health care costs, reformers should not overpromise.

The Unsurprising Surprise of Renewed Health Care Cost Inflation

Henry J. Aaron

Observers have noted that after a hiatus in the mid- and late 1990s, health care costs are once again rising fast. Like Louis Renault, the benignly corrupt police chief in *Casablanca*, who was "shocked, shocked!" that gambling was going on at Rick's Café Americain, some people are similarly stunned at the reemergence of these rapid increases. Unlike Renault, whose surprise was feigned, current observers seem genuinely startled. The more sensible reaction would be that of today's teenagers on hearing almost anything: "Well, duh!"

Health care cost inflation is not exactly new. Per capita health care expenditures have been rising 4–5% for half a century. Fluctuations have occurred, as Drew Altman and Larry Levitt's figure 1 in the previous essay shows. The recent lull was longer than others were. But the forces that have driven up costs over the long haul are, if anything, intensifying. The staggering fecundity of biomedical research is increasing, not diminishing. Rapid scientific advance always raises expenditures, even as it lowers prices. Those who think otherwise need only turn their historical eyes to automobiles, airplanes, television, and computers. In each case, massive technological advance drove down the price of services, but total outlays soared. Faulty health price statistics for many years obscured the decline in the price of achieving desired health outcomes. But recent research, well summarized by Ernst Berndt and colleagues, is on the way to removing this one anomaly.[1] Nothing, of course, has obscured the almost inexorable rise in outlays.

Other countries rein in the tendency for fully insured patients to want

Henry J. Aaron, "The Unsurprising Surprise of Renewed Health Care Cost Inflation," from *Health Affairs*, Web Exclusive, 23 January 2002, 85–87. © by Project HOPE—The People-to-People Health Foundation, Inc.

all beneficial care, regardless of cost, by subjecting hospitals or physicians or both to politically established budget limits or their functional equivalent. No such controls exist in the United States. But a variety of forces became aligned in the 1990s to temporarily attenuate the underlying tendency of fully insured patients confronting a growing menu of beneficial services to spend more and more money.

The most dramatic was the massive social experiment in private regulation of health costs known as managed care. This experiment began at the most propitious of times. Private expenditures had just completed a massive growth spurt. Health insurance premiums had also jumped and were ready to repeat their cyclical slowdown. Hospital wings echoed with unoccupied beds. Doctors' garages were filled with Mercedes Benzes. And employers were reeling under rising health care premium costs.

In this environment, managed care was well positioned to negotiate discounts from hospitals and physicians. And negotiate them they did. New pharmaceutical products and new technology shifted care from costly inpatient stays to outpatient treatments and drug therapies. And cost growth slowed.

For a few years. Meanwhile, however, new procedures continued to proliferate. New and dizzyingly costly drugs continued to emerge from clinical trials. The population continued to age. Hospitals reached their limits on discounts and struck back with demands to recontract. Managed care had picked the low-hanging fruit of easy economies. To continue holding down costs, it would have to have made palatable the denial of care that was genuinely beneficial or that patients and their physicians thought was beneficial.

Managed care couldn't do it. Perhaps, one day managed care will learn to do it. But don't bet on it. The problem is that managed care lacks political legitimacy. Managed care plans are private, often for-profit entities trying to tell sick patients who want care and physicians who think the care is necessary and who profit from providing it that it is better for the cost of that care to flow to the managed care company's bottom line than to finance medical services.

Under the best of conditions, the denial of beneficial care is difficult for employers or for their managed care agents to sustain. To make matters worse, the easy savings of managed care ended just as productivity and employment boomed. It made little sense for employers to pinch health care pennies when production dollars were abundant.

Now the situation has become genuinely nasty. The easy economies are behind us. The underlying forces driving up health care spending—biomedical advance and population aging—are intensifying. And economic growth seems to be slowing for a period of uncertain duration. Health care costs are rising fast, just as budgets, public and private, are tightening. The much-watched gross domestic product (GDP) share going to health care is likely to move up for many years to come. It is easy to see why people are worried about health cost inflation. But surprised? "Well, duh!"

Note

1   E. R. Berndt et al., "Medical Care Prices and Output," in *Handbook of Health Economics,* ed. A. J. Culyer and J. P. Newhouse (Amsterdam: Elsevier, 2000), 119–180.

The Not-So-Sad History of Medicare Cost Containment as Told in One Chart

Thomas Bodenheimer

As far as it goes, the argument of Drew Altman and Larry Levitt—that relief from private health spending growth is short-lived—is persuasive. But their history omits a crucial fact about U.S. health expenditures: While growth rates in private health spending per capita have bounced up and down, federal Medicare expenditures per enrollee have shown a consistent downward trend (figure 1).

Why? Because history shows that government regulation works. Through regulatory efforts—prospective payment of hospitals, volume performance standards for physicians, and the (unpopular but effective) Balanced Budget Act (BBA) of 1997—Medicare has slowed its rate of expenditure growth. This trend also holds true when adjusting for increases in gross domestic product (GDP) per capita.[1] Adjusting for inflation using the Consumer Price Index-Unadjusted (CPI-U), annual increases in Medicare spending per capita dropped from 11.2% for 1975–1980 to 1.8% for 1995–1999. While future Medicare expenditure growth is projected to be about 6% per year—rising above the near-zero increases of 1998 and 1999—private health spending is reaching, in Altman and Levitt's words, "double-digit rates of increase."[2] If the federal government becomes unhappy with a 6% annual Medicare growth rate, it could ratchet down this rate through a future BBA-2.

While the Medicare data can be criticized for isolating only federal spending and not including beneficiaries out-of-pocket spending, the trend is so dramatic that it cannot be ignored. Moreover, many other nations—among them Germany, Japan, Canada, and the United Kingdom

Thomas Bodenheimer, "The Not-So-Sad History of Medicare Cost Containment as Told in One Chart," from *Health Affairs*, Web Exclusive, 23 January 2002, 88–90. © 2002 by Project HOPE—The People-to-People Health Foundation, Inc.

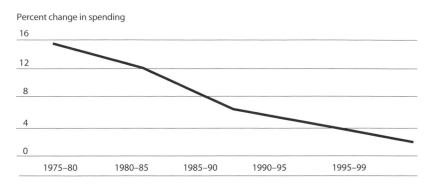

Percent change in spending

| | 1975–80 | 1980–85 | 1985–90 | 1990–95 | 1995–99 |

Figure 1. Change in Medicare Spending per Enrollee, 1975–1999. Sources: J. White, "Uses and Abuses of Long-Term Cost Estimates," *Health Affairs* (Jan/Feb 1999): 63–79; S. Heffler et al., "Health Spending Growth Up in 1999; Faster Growth Expected in the Future," *Health Affairs* (Mar/Apr 2001): 193–203; and Centers for Medicare and Medicaid Services, *Medicare: A Profile* (Baltimore: CMS, July 2000).

—have had success in dampening health care cost increases through governmental regulatory mechanisms.[3]

Painful and painless regulation. Is cost control via government regulation synonymous with rationing? Not necessarily. Cost control can be painful (denying appropriate therapies to patients) or painless.[4] Examples of painless cost control include reducing administrative waste (a product that is in abundance in the United States), cutting prices rather than quantities of services and products (particularly applicable to pharmaceuticals), and eliminating unnecessary medical interventions. Such painless cost control has the potential to save more than $100 billion per year in national health expenditures.[5]

The BBA had both painful and painless elements. The reductions in home health spending negatively affected some of the nation's most disabled citizens. Payment cuts to other providers seemed more painful to the providers than to the patients.

Could effective and long-term government regulation extend to the private health sector? In Altman and Levitt's history, two of the brief episodes decelerating the rise in private health spending were produced by governmental regulatory (or regulatory-threat) action. Public regulation of health care prices has worked in other nations.[6] There should be no disagreement about the capacity of the government to do the job. Altman and Levitt correctly identify the problem as a lack of political will.

Political barrier. One part of the political barrier is the (justified) popular desire for the latest and the best. Medicare may soon be expected to provide a permanent artificial heart pump to each of the 5 million Americans with congestive heart failure. But the political problem has a second aspect: the health care industry, whose campaign contributions assure a lucrative pricing structure. How much might Medicare pay for each of those 5 million artificial heart pumps, and how much will the surgeons installing the pumps be reimbursed? Will private insurance administrative costs continue at their 11.5% rate while Medicare is administered at 3.6%?[7] Is federal regulation of pharmaceutical prices possible without serious campaign finance reform?

In a plutocracy, Altman and Levitt's pessimism may have some justification. A true democracy—based on fundamental reform of campaign financing—would improve the chances for long-term governmental regulation of prices, elimination of unnecessary administrative costs, and reduction of inappropriate medical interventions. Altman and Levitt are right that no "easy or magic answers" are available, but the not-so-sad history of Medicare cost containment shows that solutions do exist and they do work.

Notes

1 J. White, "Uses and Abuses of Long-Term Medicare Cost Estimates," *Health Affairs* (Jan.–Feb. 1999): 63–79.
2 S. Heffler et al., "Health Spending Growth up in 1999; Faster Growth Expected in the Future," *Health Affairs* (Mar.–Apr. 2001): 193–203.
3 T. Bodenheimer and K. Grumbach, *Understanding Health Policy* (New York: McGraw-Hill, 2002), chap. 14.
4 Ibid., chap. 8.
5 S. Woolhandler and D. U. Himmelstein, "The Deteriorating Administrative Efficiency of the U.S. Health Care System," *New England Journal of Medicine* 324, no. 18 (1991): 1253–1258; and M. A. Schuster et al., "How Good Is the Quality of Health Care in the United States?" *Milbank Quarterly* 76, no. 4 (1998): 517–563.
6 Bodenheimer and Grumbach, *Understanding Health Policy,* chap. 14.
7 Heffler et al., "Health Spending Growth Up in 1999."

Medicaid and Medicare: The Unanticipated Politics of Public Insurance Programs
Lawrence D. Brown and Michael S. Sparer

Once upon a time, more or less everyone knew what genuine health reform meant. Affordable universal coverage would have the statutory shape of a European national health insurance law, or perhaps its closest American kin, Medicare. A federal enactment would create an entitlement to uniform medical benefits for all citizens, specify the funding sources that cover care thus rendered, set conditions for paying providers, and (perhaps) sketch variations on delivery arrangements. That Medicaid—a "poor people's program," means-tested, run by the states, replete with disparities in eligibility and payment levels and methods—might be, or point toward, a workable reform model was inconceivable. Persisting in this sentiment, many reformers await the next window of opportunity to enact the real thing.

In influential quarters, however—including the Democratic leadership of the U.S. Senate—Medicaid and the State Children's Health Insurance Program (SCHIP) are viewed as ready and able to sustain expansions of public health insurance that represent the nation's latest, best hope for reducing the number of uninsured people. Is the leading "poor people's program" enjoying a surprising reversal of political fortune, and if so, what might that mean? This essay contrasts aspects of the political evolution of Medicare and Medicaid and draws some challenging implications for reform.

Two Philosophies, Two Programs

Medicare and Medicaid, enacted in 1965 as Titles 18 and 19 (respectively) of that year's Social Security amendments, reflected two distinct politi-

Lawrence Brown and Michael Sparer, "Poor Program's Progress: The Unanticipated Politics of Medicaid Policy," from *Health Affairs*, vol. 22, 31–44. © 2003 by Project HOPE—The People-to-People Health Foundation, Inc.

cal philosophies and continue to do so.[1] Medicare is a universalistic program: Its 40 million beneficiaries constitute virtually all of the elderly (those age 65 and older), who are automatically entitled to its benefits. Medicaid's 40 million-plus enrollees represent only a subset of the poor (roughly two-thirds in 2002), namely, those who meet state-set eligibility rules (which are shaped in part by federal mandates) and can navigate state-administered enrollment processes.

Medicare's hospital insurance program (Part A) is financed by a social insurance trust fund. As in Social Security, employers and workers pay contributions into the trust fund over time and then (theoretically) recoup their contributions after they enter the program and start using covered services. (Medicare Part B, which covers physician services, draws on a combination of federal general revenues and premium payments by beneficiaries.) Medicaid runs on general revenues, federal and state. As in "welfare," taxpayers' dollars are collected by government and then redistributed to needy "recipients" of the public largesse.

Medicare is administered by the federal government. Not only eligibility criteria and financing policy but also the benefit package, policies governing payments to providers, and decisions about the delivery system (for instance, fee-for-service versus managed care) are determined in Washington, D.C., with no direct participation by the states. (The program delegates important decisions about coverage and payments to third-party insurers—fiscal intermediaries and carriers—and thus these national determinations do not preclude considerable regional variations that reflect local differences in wage costs and other factors.)[2] Medicaid is managed by the states. Although a framework of federal rules constrains state program administrators, they retain wide, and widening, discretion on all of the basic issues: eligibility, benefits, payments, and organization of care.

Reflections of a Political Philosophy

That these legislative twins are so decidedly unidentical is no accident. The programs' antipodal character reflected tenets of political philosophy that were widely shared among health reformers of the day (a "day" that stretched more or less seamlessly from the New Deal to the Great Society and is by no means over yet). Medicare is the preferred reform model because, so the axiom held, poor people's programs are poor programs—not only inequitable but also politically precarious. Wilbur Cohen and his colleagues worked to whittle down national health insurance (postponed under Roosevelt, stalemated under Truman, and snubbed under Eisenhower) into passable legislative shape; they sought to make Medicare both fair and formidable. Universalism promised broad, strong political support: a constituency of the elderly and their offspring that spanned social classes and income groups. Social insurance funding conferred legitimacy. Medicare was a social contract between the state and contributing citizens, who later reaped what they had sowed, not a handout.

The contractarian connotations of the trust fund carried distinct political implications: immune from the vagaries of annual appropriations that allocated general revenues in a budget process stamped by partisan and ideological fads and shifts, Medicare's resources would enjoy a stability toward which a poor people's program could never hope to aspire. Federal administration of Medicare also secured equity. States that looked askance at the elderly, government programs, or higher taxes did not get to cover fewer people and services than more "progressive" states. As befits a universal entitlement, one set of national standards applied to all major facets of Medicare in all 50 states.

Legislative Beginnings

The passage of Medicare crowned many years of patient effort to customize national health insurance as understood elsewhere to fit the stubborn exceptionalism of American politics. The enactment of Medicaid was near serendipitous, an afterthought. Wilbur Mills (then chair of the House Ways and Means Committee, which controlled the Social Security amendments), persuaded by the election of many new liberal Democrats to Congress in 1964 that new public health insurance legislation was inevitable, "proceeded to astonish policy observers" by synthesizing the existing Kerr-Mills program of federal payments to states for medical care for the poor with "Eldercare," the American Medical Association's preferred, means-tested variation on Medicare, and morphing the concoction into something called "Medicaid."[3] Reformers admired the fancy footwork and concurred that more was better, but the politics of social programs being what they were, Medicare appeared to be poised for stability and growth, while Medicaid seemed fated for chaos and perhaps retrenchment.

The evolution of the two programs over nearly four decades shows that the conventional wisdom about the political inferiority of poor people's programs—at least in the health policy arena—misses much. Medicare has indeed been stable and politically successful, but the program has seen very little expansion, whereas Medicaid has enjoyed more stability and growth than "theory" predicted.

Universalism versus Incrementalism

Medicare coverage

Political calculations limited Medicare to coverage for hospital and physician services for the elderly. These constrictions were supposedly at once necessary—to assuage opposition and get enough votes to win the hard-fought legislative battle—and transitory—once the barrier to federal financing of care was breached, additional public coverage, straight through into national health insurance, was surely imminent. The latter prognosis proved faulty, however: Medicare's benefit package remains substantially what it was in 1965 and indeed is "considerably less comprehensive than packages offered by the better employer plans."[4] Neither protracted debate nor energetic lobbying has filled such important lacunae as coverage for prescription drugs and long-term care. In 1972 the disabled and people with end-stage renal disease were made eligible for Medicare, but no comparable expansion has occurred since.

Higher-than-expected costs and attempted remedies. No sooner did implementation of Medicare commence than federal budgetmakers complained that its costs were running far higher than expected, a complaint reinforced by the high costs ("unexpected," of course) of the beneficiaries admitted in 1972. Critics of the program have cited the combination of demographic and technological trends—a steadily growing elderly population of Medicare beneficiaries lays claim to an ever expanding array of more costly and complex medical benefits—as evidence that the program is "an out-of-control entitlement that consumes too much of the federal budget and obstructs deficit reduction," that the value of the program's (stable) benefit package for the elderly has grown greatly over time, and that these endogenous forces of expansion preclude fiscally responsible additions to the current package of benefits and the corps of beneficiaries.[5]

Medicare's alleged uncontrollability is highly exaggerated. In 1983 and 1989 the program changed its methods for paying hospitals and physicians, respectively, and produced savings that eluded the private sector, a record all the more impressive because Medicare covers an older, sicker population in need of more specialized and technologically intensive services than is the case for the population at large. Between 1970 and 1998 private health insurance spending increased by a per capita average of 11% annually; Medicare's rate of growth was 10.2%.[6] More recently, provisions in the Balanced Budget Act (BBA) of 1997 sharply cut payments to hospitals, nursing homes, and home health agencies, but the howling that ensued dramatized the intensity of the cost pressures under which the program labors more than its success at holding the line.

The main exception to this pattern—the addition of catastrophic coverage to Medicare in 1988—ended as brutal proof of the rule. When the Reagan administration proposed new coverage for Medicare beneficiaries who bore exceptionally high medical expenses out of pocket, congressional Democrats "perfected" the measure by adding prescription drug benefits and other new provisions. Aiming to fund the new package without adding to the federal budget, political leaders enacted an income-related premium "surcharge" to be borne by more affluent beneficiaries. Amazed lawmakers were soon bombarded by letters and calls from angry seniors whose wrath had been stirred by organizations other than the AARP, whose soundings of constituent opinion failed to detect the danger in advance. Memorable television footage of aged protesters shouting insults and pounding on the car of Daniel Rostenkowski (then chair of the House Ways and Means Committee) generated no end of post-traumatic stress in Washington. Indeed, Ronald Vogel opined that "perhaps no other Medicare event in its 30-year history threatened members of Congress as much as the advent and demise" of the Medicare Catastrophic Coverage Act.[7] Political lessons proliferated: Sizable new benefits, if universal, were budget-busting; "responsible" budgeting and "equitable" financing meant some measure of means testing, which was a political minefield; the elderly were unreasonable and volatile; the "responsible" organizations that speak for them could not always read the political cards accurately. In 1989 Congress undid its handiwork of the year before, repealing most provisions of the new program. Ironically, much of what survived expanded Medicaid.[8]

Medicaid Coverage and Eligibility

Medicaid, which bore fewer marks than did Medicare of its creators' strategic calculations and philosophical convictions, emerged as comprehensive health coverage for people who could not afford to buy care through private means. The program has contrived to stabilize its benefits and expand its number of beneficiaries with success that is surprising in a poor people's program. The number of Medicaid clients has grown from 20 million during the 1980s to roughly 40 million in 2002.

Lacking a universalistic mandate, the program's leaders could and did consider tightening eligibility when costs rose too fast or state revenues sank too low. In the late 1960s and the 1970s, for example, both the feds and states adopted various cutting and tightening measures to cope (as in Medicare) with surprisingly rapid growth in spending. In the mid-1980s, however, the picture changed, and (in Jean Gilman's terms) the political stepchild began to emerge as Cinderella. Reductions in eligibility were seldom adopted, and most states worked to expand the ranks of eligibles. One explanation is that more penurious states could not race much farther to the bottom and more generous ones had that status because their politics made and kept them that way. But fiscal federalism was also a factor, prompting coverage expansions during good times (the feds paid most of the bill) and deterring cutbacks even in bad times (every state dollar saved meant two or three federal dollars lost).

The federal government also required expanded Medicaid coverage, demanding that states give eligibility to poor women and children at more inclusive income and age limits.[9] States duly protested these mandates, but Washington turned a deaf ear.[10] In 1996 the feds authorized Medicaid enrollment for former welfare beneficiaries, further severing Medicaid's traditional connection with welfare.

SCHIP Expansion

Medicaid served as a model, moreover, for the nation's largest publicly funded health insurance expansion since the Great Society. SCHIP, enacted in 1997, follows the Medicaid template: federal matching funds for programs in which states have wide discretion. SCHIP also allows states to reach the program's target, uninsured children who do not qualify for Medicaid, by making SCHIP an "add-on" to their Medicaid programs. These expansions may be read as no small vote of confidence in a program that has meanwhile committed growing shares of its budget to long-term care services for the indigent elderly, thus meeting needs that policy makers fear to assign to Medicare. At the end of the 1990s Medicaid and SCHIP accounted for 16% of the nation's health spending, pulling almost even with Medicare's share (18%).[11]

The despised categorical character of Medicaid invites incremental adjustments and extensions in criteria of eligibility. The feds and states alike can raise income thresholds a little here, a bit more there, as political support and financial resources permit. Such maneuvering at the margins entices and rewards policy entrepreneurs (Henry Waxman is the quintessential example), working quietly within the intricacies of the budget process to add a new group now, another benefit next time. In Waxman's own words, "Incrementalism may not get much press, but it does work."[12]

Universalism may indeed confer the power that follows the political law of large numbers, but that very fact, understood ruefully and well by policymakers, itself raises political barriers to laws incorporating further large numbers into a program whose costs are deemed uncontrollable. The vices that taint Medicaid—invidious moralism and means testing—have a virtuous correlate of no small value: strategic flexibility.

Social Insurance versus General Revenues

Medicare: Social Insurance and Fiscal Integrity

Medicare's social insurance financing has doubtless enhanced the program's legitimacy, but it has not sufficed to protect it from periodic alarms about its fiscal integrity or from intermittent "crises" over its allegedly impending bankruptcy. As Jon Oberlander points out, the trust fund mechanism makes Medicare's perceived sustainability a function of complex calculations by officially empaneled actuaries, whose computations and pronouncements cater to political Cassandras hoping to advance their agendas for change (for instance, more aggressive introduction of market forces into Medicare) by trumpeting the program's impending collapse.[13] The coalition of critics is broad indeed—"antigovernment conservatives," self-styled advocates of generational equity, and ardent antiredistributionists, conjuring up "hordes of voracious Medicare beneficiaries feasting on the hard-gotten gains of struggling, virtuous investment bankers" and the ensuing "pundit consensus" registered forcefully in public opinion.[14] In a 1995 survey only 41% of respondents knew that Medicare failed to cover prescription drugs for the elderly, but fully 70% "knew" that the program was, and had long been, in danger of bankruptcy.[15]

Over time, the opacity of the actuarial tea leaves and the opportunistic rhetorical uses to which they were put have damaged the political legitimacy that social insurance was supposed to secure. For example, pollster Celinda Lake found that people often assumed that Medicare, like Social Security, was not part of the federal budget and thus took the talk of fiscal doom as evidence that politicians were "moving money that ought to be sacrosanct and in a trust fund," that a "rotten political system . . . has raided a trust."[16] When everyone knows that Medicare is about to go broke, expansion looks utopian. When everyone accepts that its plight can be fixed only by higher taxes or more competition, deadlocks between left and right are hard to break.

Medicaid: General Revenues and Political Heat

In theory, Medicaid's reliance on general revenues ("the taxpayers' dollars") should make it a political football, and "soaring" rates of Medicaid spending have indeed generated considerable heat. This heat was most intense between 1988 and 1992, when state Medicaid budgets were rising at an average of 20.9% annually. Several variables explained these increases, including rates of medical inflation in general, the costs of absorbing newly mandated clients, increased services for people with AIDS, rising immigration, and a national economic downturn. In part, however, these rates reflected an aggravated case of the logic of expansion: state policy makers had become more aggressive than usual in laying plans to increase their federal matching shares.[17]

Managed care to the rescue. Once the dust settled—in part because Congress pulled the plug on excessively creative "scams" but also because medical inflation slowed, managed care began to yield savings in Medicaid, the economy revived, and Medicaid rolls fell—annual spending increases returned to "normal" (single-digit) figures, and Medicaid regained its status as a big-ticket state budget item that was, however, neither so vexing nor so vulnerable as to justify major reductions in eligibility and services or to derail the incremental expansions under way since the late 1980s. Medicaid rolls fell sharply in the late 1990s, to be sure, but mainly as a consequence of events external to the program itself—namely, a strong economy and, most important, welfare reform legislation of 1996, which sowed confusion by ending the automatic enrollment of public assistance clients in Medicaid, thus obliging these clients to navigate social services bureaucracies and prove their eligibility for Medicaid.

Recent budget woes. Over the past year or so Medicaid enrollment trends have shifted again, and the number of enrollees is rising dramatically, prompted by a combination of aggressive outreach and education and a weakened economy. As Medicaid costs rose 13% in 2002 while state tax revenues (in April–July 2002) fell by 10%, states put expansion on hold and worried anew about cost controls. The Kaiser Commission on Medicaid and the Uninsured reported in 2002 that 40 states had imposed controls on drug costs, 28 had reduced or frozen provider payments, 15 had increased copayments on items other than drugs, and 18 had cut eligibility in some form.[18]

Cuts are never minor to the cuttees or to those who advocate for them, but the "news" is, arguably, how marginal the contractions are, given the magnitude of the fiscal challenge. Protracted budget woes may of course call the question and test the hypothesis preferred here—namely, that Medicaid has developed constituencies of sufficient, breadth, depth, and clout to protect the program in hard times and to enlarge it when the clouds lift.

Fiscal creativity. Medicaid's reliance on general revenues raised by both states and the feds has encouraged strategic improvisations to which trust funding has been less conducive. States spending as little as 23 cents and no more than 50 cents of their own funds in each Medicaid dollar find that it pays to be creative in the search for disproportionate-share hospital (DSH) payments, federal waivers, upper payment limits, and other pots of gold. Fiscal federalism encourages "catalytic federalism": for example, states enact a small program of new coverage for non-Medicaid-eligible children and then seek a federal waiver (and accompanying federal funds) to expand it. The feds authorize Medicaid matching monies for new categories of the poor, hoping that states will find the offer too good to refuse.[19] Beyond the halcyon expansionary years of 1984–1990, moreover, lay rising reliance on federal waivers for states seeking to innovate within their Medicaid programs. Waiver politics were, and remain, a classic bargaining game in which greater state discretion is traded for enhanced public coverage and is customized, state by state, in ways Medicare cannot easily emulate.

Medicare's Endlessly Anticipated Insolvency

Meanwhile, Medicare's trust fund, cloaked in the supposedly impregnable legitimacy that inheres in an entitlement grounded in a social contract, may be losing legitimacy because its endlessly anticipated insolvency contradicts official mythology and has no clear and acceptable explanation. If Medicare is social insurance, then why do the demographics—fewer current workers making the contributions that cover the costs of the growing ranks of beneficiaries using more costly medical care over time—set the program on a road to fiscal doom from which there is (supposedly) no exit save draconian extractions from current and future workers? That Social Security itself is sometimes said to require a comparably redistributive intergenerational rescue only underscores how politically threadbare have become the contractarian arguments for social insurance in the United States.

Fee-for-Service versus Managed Care

Medicare suffers from a challenge its creators could not have foreseen in 1965: while the U.S. medical world has shifted massively to managed care arrangements, Medicare remains centered on a fee-for-service, third-party payment model that was mainstream, indeed near ubiquitous, 35 years ago. (Whether it may have retained the "right" model after all is of course an important question that cannot be pursued here.) This large antiquarian island in a sea of market forces offends conservatives who equate competition with smaller government and also troubles liberals who never liked the traditional arrangements beloved by organized medicine and want Medicare to be no less modern and innovative than the private sector. (This sense that the program is badly behind the times was one reason why the Clinton reform plan bypassed Medicare-for-all—"about 180 degrees removed from Clinton's thinking," as Ira Magaziner put it—in favor of an employer-funded system predicated on managed competition.)[20]

Medicare's Foray into Managed Care

Once both houses of Congress came under Republican control in 1996, the rush to infuse market forces and competition into Medicare soon yielded legislation (Medicare+Choice, or M+C) that stepped up federal encouragement (on the books, to little avail, since the early 1980s) for the elderly to join health maintenance organizations (HMOs). The project soon became a fiasco: HMOs sought to build market share in this revitalized market by promising elderly members benefits (prescription drug coverage in particular) absent from traditional Medicare but soon fell to quarreling with federal payers over fair payment for covering an unexpectedly expensive population. When the feds held firm (the plans were selecting preferred risks, said officials from the Centers for Medicare and Medicaid Services [CMS, formerly known as HCFA], and falling short on the management of care to boot), plans began abandoning the Medicare market. Many seniors found themselves without the promised extras, indeed without HMO coverage at all, and the well-publicized upheavals added fuel to a growing backlash that did nothing to endear managed care to Medicare's many stakeholders.[21] Between 1998 and 2001 the number of managed care plans participating in Medicare+Choice dropped roughly by half (from 346 to 179), and managed care penetration among beneficiaries fell to 14%—a rate that the Congressional Budget Office forecasts will hit a mere 18% of beneficiaries in 2011.[22]

Medicaid's More Successful Managed Care Venture

Medicaid has, for better or worse, modernized itself into managed care more adroitly than has Medicare. One possible explanation, of course, is that poor people, who do not vote much and lack AARP-like organizations to defend them, are easier to "force" into managed care than are the elderly. States had to win federal waiver authority to proceed with Medicaid managed care, however, and, under intense scrutiny from HCFA/CMS, state policymakers averred that they were designing managed care that would expand access and improve quality even as it slowed the growth of costs. States did not (for the most part) slash payment rates dramatically in anticipation of imminent savings, although they did impose potent regulatory controls on health plans entering the Medicaid market.

Nowhere has Medicaid managed care been an easy ride, and the misadventures of M+C—the plans' rush to sew up market share, the misrepresentations in marketing to befuddled enrollees, indignation over the more-expensive-to-serve-than-predicted clientele, battles between plans and government over fair rates, the huffy exits of aggrieved plans, and jilted enrollees scrambling for new plans or providers—have all surfaced, in varying degrees, in Medicaid managed care programs. On the whole, however, the interplay of the feds and states in Medicaid has more successfully installed midcourse corrections into managed care for the 56% of clients who are in it than has the stalemated byplay between the feds and plans that governs managed care for its 14% of Medicare beneficiaries.

The difference derives precisely from Medicaid's initially suspect character as a joint federal-state endeavor. Medicaid combines a framework of federal rules and guidance with 50 varieties of state-plan relations. Medicare combines voluminous rules with much more constricted responsiveness to variations in state politics and regional markets. Moreover, having moved down the road to managed care for their Medicaid clients, states, unlike the feds, cannot call the plans' bluff, knowing that a fee-for-service sector stands ready to accept refugees. Medicaid managed care arose from the conviction that the fee-for-service system gave inadequate access and quality at excessive cost. If states cannot after all buy good care cheaply, they must either go back to painful wrestling with fee-for-service, raise rates (and refine regulations) sufficiently to make the managed care market work, or—the emerging strategy of choice—negotiate acceptable arrangements with managed care plans formed by safety net institutions that have long served as providers of last resort for the poor.

Medicare beneficiaries, unique among insured U.S. citizens (although entirely typical of citizens covered by the national health insurance systems of other Western nations), can fall back on yesterday's mainstream should modernization by means of managed care flop. Having acknowledged that yesterday's mainstream had grown indefensible for Medicaid's patients and purchasers alike, states have little choice but to contrive somehow to manage the care of the poor.

The Poor People's Program and Policy Reform

Few would deny that Medicare is a great and good program or that Medicaid retains both a weighty cultural burden of welfare medicine and disturbingly low adult eligibility levels in many states. The point of this comparative sketch of the political evolution of the two programs is not to bury Medicare or praise Medicaid as public programs but rather to challenge inherited reform models.

The perpetual perils of comprehensive health reform, reenacted vividly a decade ago by the Clinton health plan, suggest that the universalism in affordable coverage may lie beyond the polity's capacity any time soon: 85% of the population has coverage; the 15% that lack it are unorganized and uncohesive; redistributive politics are tough in the best of times; the lingering antigovernmental ethos that set in 35 years ago continues to make the going that much rougher; and the consoling myth that the safety net provides all of the care that those without coverage really need stifles any sense of popular urgency around the issue.

The fabled connections between universalism and strong political constituencies have, furthermore, grown strained and murky. The political strength of the nation's elderly, their offspring, health care providers, medical suppliers, and other Medicare contractors registers far more potently in defensive maneuvers to block threatening changes than in expansions of benefits or beneficiaries.[23]

Medicaid's Broad Constituency

Meanwhile, and contrary to first impressions, Medicaid's constituency has grown well beyond the nation's welfare poor. In 1974 Robert Stevens and Rosemary Stevens regretted "a lack of clarity about what Medicaid was and for whom it was created" but added that this "catch-all program" with ambiguous boundaries had expansionary potential that might yield a constituency "at least as wide as that of Medicare."[24] This forecast has proved prescient: a sizable corps of physicians, hospitals, community health centers, and public health clinics, including but not limited to those that constitute the safety net, have tangible interests not only in what Medicaid pays but also in whom it covers and thus shelters from the rolls of charity care patients. The indigent elderly (and those in the process of spending down to become so) plus the nursing homes and home health agencies that serve them fight contractions in America's major long-term care program. A range of managed care plans has joined (and then sometimes left) the crowd of Medicaid's stakeholders. Fifty states, and the elected officials who enjoy showering federal benefits on them, perpetually ponder the seductions of 50 or more federal cents on each Medicaid dollar (half the states get a federal match of 60% or more, while 10, including the District of Columbia, get upward of 70%). Medicaid permits members of Congress "to claim credit for providing benefits while shifting half of the cost to the states."[25] Political liberals see realized in Medicaid the powerful (albeit nonuniversalistic) principle of targeting: to each according to his or her needs.

The needs Medicaid meets have steadily expanded and now stretch well beyond the impoverished women and children with whom the program is popularly identified. Roughly two-thirds of Medicaid spending serves the aged, blind, and disabled, who are about one-quarter of its beneficiaries. The equation of poor people's programs with poor programs failed to capture how heterogeneous and capacious the categories of entitlement would become as the politics of social policy played on.

Universalism and U.S. Political Culture

A glance at national health insurance in other nations suggests that universalism has crucial moral underpinnings. Other Western societies accept as a kind of normative axiom that care is not enough, that basic human dignity would be offended if any citizen declined to seek medical care for fear of the financial consequences of doing so or faced financial stress as a consequence of getting care. This simple but indispensable conviction has so far failed to register strongly in U.S. political culture, and there are no current signs that it is beginning to do so. A massive political and ideological shift like those of 1932 and 1964 could change this prognosis overnight, but in the meantime sustaining and stretching incremental extensions of coverage to means-tested categories of the uninsured may be the nation's best bet for shrinking the number of uninsured Americans to the point at which employer buy-ins and kindred measures may supply coverage for those nonpoor uninsured whom Medicaid may never reach.

Stigma of Social Insurance

Even if the political stars aligned to produce a universal, national entitlement to health coverage, social insurance financing is unlikely to confer the social legitimacy and political insulation the founders of Social Security and Medicare cherished. Social insurance has served this and other countries very well for many years, and if magic wands were available, what rational actor would not cheerfully install the French or German health care system in place of the U.S. status quo? Years of apocalyptic predictions that Medicare (like Social Security) totters near bankruptcy, will not "be there" when today's contributors retire, and can be salvaged only by Sisyphean lifting by current workers have, however, stigmatized social insurance along with the "t" word ("taxes") in general. Although no single source—employer mandates, social insurance, or general revenues—will do the whole job, the latter will probably have to supply much of the money needed to cover 40 million uninsured people. (The French, for example, have steadily supplemented their "Bismarckian" social insurance–funded health regime with infusions of general revenues that tap a broader

89

range of wealth.) Reformers might want to scrutinize more closely than is customary how the feds and states combine to steer the political economy of fiscal federalism in Medicaid, which runs entirely on taxpayers' closely watched dollars.

Universal Entitlement with Regional Variations

Even if a universalistic entitlement and social insurance funds proved to be politically feasible, a centrally run program with uniform national rules is unlikely to be the preferred administrative vehicle. The states have grown too prominent and too powerful not to insist on wide spheres of discretion, and managed care's sensitivity to local market settings precludes dispelling all disparities. For public managers the trick will be to fashion a set of national rules that protects the interests of the insured without proscribing state and regional variations (in organizational arrangements, payment provisions, perhaps supplemental benefits, and more) that do not cross the line into objectionable inequities. Canadian federalism offers one instructive approach: 10 distinct provincial systems linked by acceptance of a short list of national principles that set conditions for the sharing of provincial costs with the central government. The accumulation of federal-state accommodations in Medicaid, and especially the long yet underexamined saga of federal waivers to support state innovations in that program, doubtless suggest further lessons.

Health reform in the 21st century will not resemble the New Deal or Great Society Oldsmobile, much less their Cadillac. Pondering the surprising evolution of Medicaid and the reasons why it is not so poor a program after all may help reorient a policy debate that risks losing its way within nostalgic mists. The succinct "lessons" are these: add groups by raising income thresholds incrementally; use federal-state matching to catalyze creative use of general revenues; experiment with managed care (and then labor to get it out of the theoretical clouds and onto firm institutional ground); try to get rates of uninsurance among children down to low single digits; try to add family coverage; seek political openings to narrow eligibility gaps; and work harder to enroll eligible people. Might one see coming into view, albeit dimly, a model of universal coverage—inelegant, impure, and replete with disparities to be sure—that may be sufficiently distinct to fit America's stubborn exceptionalism?

Notes

1　See T. R. Marmor, *The Politics of Medicare*, 2d ed. (New York: Aldine de Gruyter, 2000) (a modestly dubbed "second edition" that adds to the first several new chapters indispensable for understanding the program); and J. Oberlander, *Political Life of Medicare* (Chicago: University of Chicago Press, 2003). Our main sources for Medicaid are R. Stevens and R. Stevens, *Welfare Medicine in America: A Case Study of Medicaid* (New York: Free Press, 1974); M. Sparer, *Medicaid and the Limits of Health Reform* (Philadelphia: Temple University Press, 1996); and J. D. Gilman, *Medicaid and the Costs of Federalism, 1984–1992* (New York: Garland, 1998). Gilman admirably addresses, from a different slant, many of the questions we tackle here.

2　See B. C. Vladeck, "The Political Economy of Medicare," *Health Affairs* (Jan.–Feb. 1999): 22–36.

3　E. D. Berkowitz, *America's Welfare State: From Roosevelt to Reagan* (Baltimore: Johns Hopkins University Press, 1999), 173.

4　R. M. Ball, "Reflections on How Medicare Came About," in *Medicare: Preparing for the Challenges of the Twenty-first Century*, ed. R. D. Reischauer et al. (Washington: National Academy of Social Insurance, 1998), 36.

5　See Marmor, *The Politics of Medicare*, 96, 127.

6　Ibid., 128; and Henry J. Kaiser Family Foundation, *Medicare Chart Book*, 2d ed. (Menlo Park, Calif.: Kaiser Family Foundation, fall 2001), 30.

7　R. J. Vogel, *Medicare: Issues in Political Economy* (Ann Arbor: University of Michigan Press, 1999), 75.

8　R. Himelfarb, *Catastrophic Politics: The Rise and Fall of the Medicare Catastrophic Coverage Act of 1988* (University Park: Pennsylvania State University Press, 1995); and Marmor, *The Politics of Medicare*, 110–113.

9　See Gilman, *Medicaid and the Costs of Federalism*, 59–72, for measures expanding eligibility and benefits.

10　Ibid., 103–104.

11　Kaiser Family Foundation, *Medicare Chart Book*, 23.

12　Gilman, *Medicaid and the Costs of Federalism*, 141.

13　Oberlander, *Political Life of Medicare*, chap. 4.

14　T. Skocpol, "Pundits, People, and Medicare Reform," in *Medicare*, ed. Reischauer et al., 23, 25; Marmor, *The Politics of Medicare*, 124; and Vladeck, "The Political Economy of Medicare," 26.

15　F. E. Mebane, *Medicare Politics: Exploring the Roles of Medical Coverage, Political Information, and Political Participation* (New York: Garland, 2000), 45.

16　"View by Celinda Lake," in *Medicare*, ed. Reischauer et al., 308, 312.

17　For a discussion of state financing stratagems, see Gilman, *Medicaid and the Costs of Federalism*, 155–183.

18　Kaiser Commission on Medicaid and the Uninsured, "State Budgets under Stress: How Are States Planning to Reduce the Growth in Medicaid Costs?" (Washington: Kaiser Commission, 30 July 2002); and *Medicaid Spending Growth: Results from a 2002 Survey* (Washington: Kaiser Commission, September 2002).

19   L. D. Brown and M. S. Sparer, "Window Shopping: State Health Reform Politics in the 1990s," *Health Affairs* (Jan.–Feb. 2001): 50–67.

20   H. Johnson and D. S. Broder, *The System: The American Way of Politics at the Breaking Point* (Boston: Little, Brown, 1996), 398.

21   N. M. DeParle, "As Good as It Gets? The Future of Medicare+Choice," *Journal of Health Politics, Policy and Law* (June 2002): 495–512.

22   Kaiser Family Foundation, *Medicare Chart Book*, 51–52.

23   Vladeck, "The Political Economy of Medicare," 26–31.

24   Stevens and Stevens, *Welfare Medicine*, 349, 51–52. On the breadth of Medicaid's coalition, also see Gilman, *Medicaid and the Costs of Federalism*, 95, 146.

25   Gilman, *Medicaid and the Costs of Federalism*, 188.

PART II

Managed Care, Markets, and Rationing

Bedside Manna
Deborah Stone

For more than 150 years, American medicine aspired to an ethical ideal of the separation of money from medical care. Medical practice was a money-making proposition, to be sure, and doctors were entrepreneurs as well as healers. But the lodestar that guided professional calling and evoked public trust was the idea that at the bedside, clinical judgment should be untainted by financial considerations.

Although medicine never quite lived up to that ideal, the new regime of managed care health insurance is an epic reversal of the principle. Today, insurers deliberately try to influence doctors' clinical decisions with money—either the prospect of more of it or the threat of less. What's even more astounding is that this manipulation of medical judgment by money is no longer seen in policy circles as a corruption of science or a betrayal of the doctor-patient relationship. Profit-driven medical decision making is extolled as the path to social responsibility, efficient use of resources, and even medical excellence.

How did such a profound cultural revolution come about? What does the new culture of medicine mean for health care? And where does it leave the welfare state and the culture of solidarity on which it rests when the most respected and essential caregivers in our society are encouraged to let personal financial reward dictate how they pursue patients' welfare?

Money and Medicine

Before the mid-19th century, the business relationship between doctors and patients was simple: the patient paid money in exchange for the doc-

Deborah Stone, "Bedside Manna," from *The American Prospect*, vol. 8, 42–48, March/April 1997. © 1997 by The American Prospect, Inc. Reprinted by permission of Deborah Stone and the publisher.

tor's advice, skill, and medicines. However, to win acceptance as professionals and be perceived as something more than commercial salesmen, doctors needed to persuade the public that they were acting out of knowledge and altruism rather than self-interest and profit. Organized medicine built a system of formal education, examinations, licensing, and professional discipline, all meant to assure that doctors' recommendations were based on medical science and the needs of the patient, rather than profit seeking.

In theory, this system eliminated commercial motivation from medicine by selecting high-minded students, acculturating them during medical training, and enforcing a code of ethics that put patients' interests first. In practice, medicine remained substantially a business, and no one behaved more like an economic cartel than the American Medical Association. The system of credentialing doctors eventually eliminated most alternative healers and, by limiting the supply of doctors, enhanced the profitability of doctoring. Nonetheless, medical leaders espoused the ideal and justified these and other market restrictions as necessary to protect patients' health, not doctors' incomes.

It took the growth of health insurance to create a system in which a doctor truly did not need to consider patients' financial means in weighing their clinical needs, so long as the patient was insured. As Columbia University historian David Rothman has shown, private health insurance was advertised to the American middle class on the promise that it would neutralize financial considerations when people needed medical care. Blue Cross ads hinted darkly that health insurance meant not being treated like a poor person—not having to use the public hospital and not suffering the indignity of a ward. Quality of medical care, the ads screamed between the lines, was indeed connected to money, but health insurance could sever the connection.

By 1957, the AMA's Principles of Medical Ethics forbade a doctor to "dispose of his services under terms or conditions that tend to interfere with or impair the free and complete exercise of his medical judgment or skill." This statement was the apotheosis of the ethical ideal of separating clinical judgment from money. It symbolized the long struggle to make doctoring a scientific and humane calling rather than a commercial enterprise, at least in the public's eyes if not always in actual fact. But the AMA never acknowledged that fee-for-service payment, the dominant arrangement and the only payment method it approved at the time, might itself "interfere with" medical judgment.

Meanwhile, as costs climbed in the late 1960s, research began to show that fee-for-service payment seemed to induce doctors to hospitalize their patients more frequently compared to other payment methods such as flat salaries, and that professional disciplinary bodies rarely, if ever, monitored financial conflicts of interest. Other research showed that the need for medical services in any given population was quite elastic, often a matter of discretion, and that doctors could diagnose enough needs for their own and their hospitals' services to keep everybody running at full throttle.

Still, the cultural premise of these controversies expressed a clear moral imperative: ethical medicine meant money should not be a factor in medical decision making. The new findings about money's influence on medicine were accepted as muck that needed raking. Occasional exposés of medical incentive schemes—for example, bonuses from drug and device companies for prescribing their products or kickbacks for referrals to diagnostic testing centers—were labeled "fraud and abuse" and branded as outside the pale of normal, ethical medicine.

The Path Not Taken

Sooner or later, the ideal of medical practice untainted by financial concerns had to clash with economic reality. Everything that goes into medical care is a resource with a cost, and people's decisions about using resources are always at least partly influenced by cost. By the 1970s, with health care spending hitting 9% of the gross national product (GNP) and costs for taxpayers and employers skyrocketing, America perceived itself to be in a medical cost crisis. Doctors and hospitals, however, resisted cost control measures. By the late 1980s, neither the medical profession, the hospitals, the insurers, nor the government had managed to reconcile the traditional fee-for-service system with cost control, even though the number of people without health insurance grew steadily.

During these decades, a pervasive antigovernment sentiment and a resurgence of laissez-faire capitalism on the intellectual right combined to push the United States toward market solutions to its cost crisis. Other countries with universal public-private health insurance systems have watched their spending rise, too, driven by the same underlying forces of demographics and technology. But unlike the United States, they rely on organized cooperation and planning to contain costs rather than on influencing individual doctors with financial punishment or reward. Some national health systems pay each doctor a flat salary, which eliminates the financial incentive to overtreat, though it might create a mild incentive to undertreat. Systems with more nearly universal health insurance schemes also eliminate expensive competition between insurers, because there is no outlay for risk selection, marketing, or case-by-case pretreatment approval, and far less administrative expense generally.

Countries with comprehensive systems typically plan technology acquisition by doctors and hospitals to moderate one of the chief sources of medical inflation. Most also limit the total supply of doctors, or of specialists, through higher-education policy. They may restrict doctors' geographic location in order to meet needs of rural areas and dampen excess medical provision in cities. Most countries with universal systems have some kind of global budget cap. But the difficult medical trade-offs within that budget constraint are made by clinicians under broad general guidelines, and not on the basis of commercial incentives to individual doctors facing individual patients. Significantly, although government is usually a guiding force in these systems, planning is done by councils or commissions that represent and cooperate with doctors, hospitals, other professions, medical suppliers, insurers, unions, and employer associations.

The distinctive feature of the emerging American way of cost control is our reliance on market competition and personal economic incentive to govern the system. For the most part, such incentives are contrived by insurers. In practice, that has meant insurers have far more power in our system than in any other, and it has meant that they insert financial considerations into medical care at a level of detail and personal control unimaginable in any other country.

Reconfiguring the Role of Money

The theorists of market reform reversed the traditional norm that the doctor-patient relationship should be immune to pecuniary interests. Law professor Clark Havighurst, HMO-advocate Paul Ellwood, and economist Alain Enthoven and their disciples celebrated the power of financial motivation to economize in medical care. In the process, they elaborated a moral justification for restoring money to a prominent place in the doctor's mind.

In what is probably the single most important document of the cultural revolution in medical care, Alain Enthoven began his 1978 Shattuck Lecture to the Massachusetts Medical Society by explaining why he, an economist, should be giving this distinguished lecture instead of a doctor. The central problem of medicine, he said, was no longer simply how to cure the sick, eliminate quackery, and achieve professional excellence, but rather how people could "most effectively use their resources to promote the health of the population." Enthoven dismissed government regulation as ineffective. The key issue was "how to motivate physicians to use hospital and other resources economically." It was time, he concluded, for doctors to look beyond the biological sciences as they crafted the art of medicine, and to draw on cost-effectiveness analysis.

In Enthoven's vision, researchers would incorporate cost-benefit calculations into clinical guidelines; health plans would give doctors incentives to follow these guidelines; and if patients were allowed to shop for plans in an open market, the most efficient plans would win greater market share. We could succeed in "Cutting Costs without Cutting the Quality of Care," as the title of his lecture promised. The ultimate safeguard against financial temptations to skimp on quality or quantity of care, according to Enthoven, was "the freedom of the dissatisfied patient to change doctors or health plan."

In market theory, consumers are the disciplinary force that keeps producers honest. In applying classical market theory to medicine, theorists such as Havighurst and Enthoven confused consumer with payer. By the late 1970s, when medical care was paid for by private and public insurers or by charity, patient and payer were seldom the same person.

Precisely this ambiguity about the identity of the consumer gave market rhetoric its political appeal. It papered over a deep political conflict over who would control medical care—insurers, patients, doctors, or government. Market imagery suggested to insurers and employers that they, as purchasers of care, would gain control, while it suggested to patients that they, as consumers of care, would be sovereign. For a brief while in the 1970s and 1980s, the women's health movement and a Ralph Nader-inspired health consumer movement adopted market rhetoric, too, thinking that consumer sovereignty would empower patients vis-à-vis their doctors. For their part, many doctors came to accept the introduction of explicit financial incentives into their clinical practice, because, they were told, it was the only alternative to the bogey of government regulation. ("Health care spending will inevitably be brought under control," warned Enthoven in his Shattuck Lecture. "Control could be effected voluntarily by physicians in a system of rational incentives, or by direct economic regulation by the government.")

Enthoven's early approach relied only partly on the discipline of personal reward or punishment for doctors. He also advocated doing more research on cost-effectiveness and educating of doctors to make better use of scarce resources. And like Ellwood, Havighurst, and most advocates of market competition in medicine, Enthoven recognized the differences between medicine and ordinary commerce when he argued that competition had to be regulated in order to limit opportunism and enable patients to discipline insurance plans. But the heavy overlay of regulation originally envisioned by Enthoven and others was not established. While some HMOs have been more diligent than others in bringing quality and outcomes research to bear on medical practice, monetary incentives have become the paramount form of cost discipline.

Remaking the Doctor as Entrepreneur

Today, financial incentives on doctors are reversed. Instead of the general incentives of fee-for-service medicine to perform more services and procedures, contractual arrangements between payers and doctors now exert financial pressures to do less. These pressures affect every aspect of the doctor-patient relationship: how doctors and patients choose each other, how many patients a doctor accepts, how much time he or she spends with them, what diagnostic tests the doctor orders, what referrals the doctor makes, what procedures to perform, which of several potentially beneficial therapies to administer, which of several potentially effective drugs to prescribe, whether to hospitalize a patient, when to discharge a patient, and when to give up on a patient with severe illness.

In most HMOs, doctors are no longer paid by one simple method, such as salary, fee-for-service, or capitation (a fixed fee per patient per year). Instead, the doctor's pay is linked to other medical expenditures through a system of multiple accounts, pay withholding, rebates, bonuses, and penalties. Health plans typically divide their budget into separate funds for primary care services, specialists, hospital care, laboratory tests, and prescription drugs. The primary care doctors receive some regular pay, which may be based on salary, capitation, or fee-for-service, but part of their pay is calculated after the fact, based on the financial condition of the other funds. And there's the rub.

Studies of HMOs by Alan Hillman of the University of Pennsylvania found that two-thirds of HMOs routinely withhold a part of each primary care doctor's pay. Of the plans that withhold, about a third withhold less than 10% of the doctor's pay and almost half withhold between 11 and 20%. A few withhold even more. These "withholds" are the real financial stick of managed care, because doctors are told they may eventually receive all, part, or none of their withheld pay. In some HMOs, the rebate a doctor receives depends solely on his or her own behavior—whether he or she sent too many patients to specialists, ordered too many tests, or had too many patients in the hospital. In other plans, each doctor's rebate is tied to the performance of a larger group of doctors. In either case, doctors are vividly aware that a significant portion of their pay is tied to their willingness to hold down the care they dole out.

Withholding pay is itself a strong influence on doctors' clinical decisions, but other mechanisms tighten the screws even further. Forty percent of HMOs make primary care doctors pay for patients' lab tests out of their own payments or from a combined fund for primary care doctors and outpatient tests. Many plans (around 30% in Hillman's original survey) impose penalties on top of withholding, and they have invented penalties with Kafkaesque relish: increasing the amount withheld from a doctor's pay in the following year, decreasing the doctor's regular capitation rate, reducing the amount of rebate from future surpluses, or even putting liens on a doctor's future earnings. A doctor's pay in different pay periods can commonly vary by 20 to 50% as a result of all these incentives, according to a 1994 survey sponsored by the Physician Payment Review Commission.

Of course, not all HMOs provide financial incentives that reward doctors for denying necessary care. In principle, consumers could punish managed care plans that restricted clinical freedoms, and doctors could refuse to work for them. But as insurers merge and a few gain control of large market shares, and as one or two HMOs come to dominate a local market, doctors and patients may not have much choice about which ones to join. The theorists' safeguards may prove largely theoretical.

In the early managed-market theory of Enthoven and others, the doctor was supposed to make clinical decisions on the basis of cost-effectiveness analysis. That would mean considering the probability of "success" of procedure, the cost of care for each patient, and the benefit to society of spending resources for this treatment on this patient compared to spending them in some other way. But in the new managed care payment systems, financial incentives do not push doctors to think primarily about cost-effectiveness but rather to think about the effect of costs on their own income. Instead of asking themselves whether a procedure is medically necessary for a patient or cost-effective for society, they are led to ask whether it is financially tolerable for themselves. Conscientious doctors may well try to use their knowledge of cost-effectiveness studies to help them make the difficult rationing decisions they are forced to make, but the financial incentives built into managed care do not in themselves encourage anything but personal income maximization. Ironically, managed care returns doctors to the role of salesmen—but now they are rewarded for selling fewer services, not more.

Who Cares?

Because doctors in managed care often bear some risk for the costs of patient care, they face some of the same incentives that induce commercial health insurance companies to seek out healthy customers and avoid sick or potentially sick ones. In an article in *Health Affairs*, David Blumenthal, chief of health policy research and development at Massachusetts General Hospital, explained why his recent bonuses had varied:

> Last spring I received something completely unexpected: a check for $1,200 from a local health maintenance organization (HMO) along with a letter congratulating me for spending less than predicted on their 100 or so patients under my care. I got no bonus the next quarter because several of my patients had elective arthroscopies for knee injuries. Nor did I get a bonus from another HMO, because three of their 130 patients under my care had been hospitalized over the previous six months, driving my actual expenditures above expected for this group.

Such conscious linking of specific patients to paychecks is not likely to make doctors think that their income depends on how cost-effectively they practice, as market theory would have it. Rather, they are likely to conclude, with some justification, that their income depends on the luck of the draw—how many of their patients happen to be sick in expensive ways. The payment system thus converts each sick patient, even each illness, into a financial liability for doctors, a liability that can easily change their attitude toward sick patients. Doctors may come to resent sick people and to regard them as financial drains.

Dr. Robert Berenson, who subsequently became co–medical director of an HMO, gave a moving account of this phenomenon in the *New Republic* in 1987. An elderly woman was diagnosed with inoperable cancer shortly after she enrolled in a Medicare managed care plan with him as her primary care doctor, and her bills drained his bonus account: "At a time when the doctor-patient relationship should be closest, concerned with the emotions surrounding death and dying, the HMO payment system introduced a divisive factor. I ended up resenting the seemingly unending medical needs of the patient and the continuing demands placed on me by her distraught family. To me, this Medicare beneficiary had effectively become a 'charity patient.' "

Thus do the financial incentives under managed care spoil doctors' relationships to illness and to people who are ill. Illness becomes something for the doctor to avoid rather than something to treat, and sick patients become adversaries rather than subjects of compassion and intimacy.

Here is also the source of the most profound social change wrought by the American approach to cost containment. Health insurance marketing from the 1930s to the 1950s promised subscribers more reliable access to high-quality care than they could expect as charity patients. But as it is now evolving, managed care insurance will soon render all its subscribers charity patients. By tying doctors' income to the cost of each patient, managed care lays bare what was always true about health insurance: the kind of care sick people get, indeed whether they get any care at all, depends on the generosity of others.

Insurance, after all, is organized generosity. It always redistributes from those who don't get sick to those who do. Classic indemnity insurance, by pooling risk anonymously, masking redistribution, and making the users of care relatively invisible to the nonusers, created the illusion that care was free and that no one had to be generous for the sick to be treated. It was a system designed to induce generosity on the part of doctors and fellow citizens. But managed care insurance, to the extent it exposes and highlights the costs to others of sick people's care, is calculated to dampen generosity.

Putting the Doctor-Businessman to Work

The insulation of medical judgment from financial concerns was always partly a fiction. The ideal of the doctor as free of commercial influence was elaborated by a medical profession that sought to expand its market and maintain its political power and autonomy. Now, the opposite ideal—

the doctor as ethical businessman whose financial incentives and professional calling mesh perfectly—is promoted in the service of a different drive to expand power and markets.

Corporate insurers use this refashioned image of the doctor to recruit both doctors and patients. The new image has some appeal to doctors, in part because it acknowledges that they need and want to make money in a way the old ethical codes didn't, and in part because it conveys a (false) sense of independence at a time when clinical autonomy is fast eroding. Through financial incentives and requirements for patients to get their treatments and tests authorized in advance, insurers are taking clinical decisions out of doctors' hands. Hospital length-of-stay rules, drug formularies (lists of drugs a plan will cover), and exclusive contracts with medical-device suppliers also reduce doctors' discretion.

In contrast to this reality of diminished clinical authority, images of the doctor as an entrepreneur, as a risk taker, as "the 'general manager' of his patient's medical care" (that's Enthoven's sobriquet in his Shattuck Lecture) convey a message that clinical doctors are still in control. If they practice wisely, in accord with the dictates of good, cost-effective medicine, they will succeed at raising their income without cutting quality. HMOs have long exploited this imagery of business heroism to recruit physicians. Here's Stephen Moore, then medical director of United Health Care, explaining to doctors in the *New England Journal of Medicine* in 1979 how this new type of HMO would help them fulfill "their desire to control costs" while keeping government regulation at bay:

> Incentives encourage the primary-care physician to give serious consideration to his new role as the coordinator and financial manager of all medical care. . . . Because accounts and incentives exist for each primary-care physician, the physician's accountability is not shared by other physicians, even among partners in a group practice. . . . Each physician is solely responsible for the efficiency of his own health care system. . . . In essence, then, the individual primary-care physician becomes a one-man HMO.

The image of entrepreneur suggests that doctors' success depends on their skill and acumen as managers. It plays down the degree to which their financial success and ability to treat all patients conscientiously depend on the mix of sick and costly patients in their practices and the practices of other doctors with whom they are made to share risks.

The once negative image of doctor-as-businessman has been recast to appeal to patients, too, as insurers, employers, and Medicare and Medicaid programs try to persuade patients to give up their old-style insurance and move into managed care plans. Doctors, the public has been told by all the crisis stories of the past two decades, have been commercially motivated all along. They exploited the fee-for-service system and generous health insurance policies to foist unnecessary and excessive "Cadillac" services onto patients, all to line their own pockets. Patients, the story continues, have been paying much more than necessary to obtain adequate, good-quality medical care. But now, under the good auspices of insurers, doctors' incentives will be perfectly aligned with the imperatives of scientifically proven medical care, doctors will be converted from bad businessmen to good, and patients will get more value for their money.

If patients knew how much clinical authority was actually stripped from their doctors in managed care plans, they might be more reluctant to join. The marketing materials of managed care plans typically exaggerate doctors' autonomy. They tell potential subscribers that their primary care doctor has the power to authorize any needed services, such as referral to specialists, hospitalization, X-rays, lab tests, and physical therapy. Doctors in these marketing materials "coordinate" all care, "permit" patients to see specialists, and "decide" what care is medically necessary. Meanwhile, the actual contracts often give HMOs the power to authorize medically necessary services, and more important, to define what services fall under the requirements for HMO approval.

In managed care brochures, doctors not only retain their full professional autonomy, but under the tutelage of management experts, they work magic with economic resources. Through efficient management, they actually increase the value of the medical care dollar. "Because of our expertise in managing health care," a letter to Medicare beneficiaries from the Oxford Medicare Advantage plan promised, "Oxford is able to give you *100% of your Medicare benefits and much, much more*" [emphasis in original]. Not a word in these sales materials about the incentives for doctors to deny expensive procedures and referrals, nor in some cases, the "gag clauses" that prevent doctors from telling patients about treatments a plan won't cover.

In an era when employers and governments are reducing their financial commitments to workers and citizens, the image of the doctor as efficient manager is persuasive rhetoric to mollify people who have come to expect certain benefits. To lower their costs, employers are cutting back on fringe benefits and shifting jobs to part-time and contract employees, to whom they have no obligation to provide health insurance. The federal and state governments are similarly seeking to cut back the costs of Medicare and Medicaid. The image of the doctor as an efficient manager—someone who can actually increase the value to patients of the payer's reduced payments—helps gain beneficiaries' assent to reductions in their benefits. Thus, the cultural icon of doctor-as-businessman has become a source of power for employers and governments as they cut back private and public social welfare commitments.

The old cultural ideal of pure clinical judgment without regard to costs or profits always vibrated with unresolved tensions. It obscured the reality that doctoring was a business as well as a profession and that medical care costs money and consumes resources. But now that commercial managed care has turned doctors into entrepreneurs who maximize profits by minimizing care, the aspirations of the old ideal are worth reconsidering.

In trying to curb costs, we should not economize in ways that subvert the essence of medical care or the moral foundations of community. There is something worthwhile about the idea of medicine as a higher calling with a healing mission, dedicated to patients' welfare above doctors' incomes and committed to serving people on the basis of their needs, not their status. If we want compassionate medical care, we have to structure both medical care and health insurance to inspire compassion. We must find a way, as other countries have, to insure everybody on relatively equal terms, and thus divorce clinical decisions from the patient's pocketbook and the doctor's personal profit. This will require systems that control expenditures, as other countries do, without making doctor and patient financial adversaries. There is no perfect way to reconcile cost containment with clinical autonomy, but surely, converting the doctor into an entrepreneur is the most perverse strategy yet attempted.

Must Good HMOs Go Bad?
The Commercialization of Prepaid Group Health Care
Robert Kuttner

Prepaid group health care began in the 1940s as an insurgent, even radical form of medicine. At the time, few Americans had health insurance. The early programs would later be called group or staff models—closed systems with salaried doctors and an emphasis on prevention. The members sacrificed an often hypothetical freedom of choice for security and continuity of care. The doctors sacrificed independent, fee-for-service practice for a stable salary, a collegial setting, and a social ethic. Such plans were fiercely resisted by organized medicine.[1,2]

The shift in prepaid group health care from an insurgent social movement to the most entrepreneurial and occasionally ruthless part of the health care system represents a stunning reversal. The turning point was in the early 1970s, when then President Richard Nixon rebaptized prepaid group health care plans as health maintenance organizations (HMOs), with legislation that provided for federal endorsement, certification, and assistance. HMOs today are widely seen as entrepreneurial agents of cost containment. The proportion of HMO members enrolled in for-profit loans has increased from 12% in 1981 to about 62% today.[3] Nearly three HMOs in four are now for-profit, shareholder-owned plans.[4]

Whereas organized medicine once opposed group health as socialistic, medical societies now resist excessive corporate meddling by nonclinicians running HMOs. Today's cost cutting is driven jointly by the demands of payers (employers and governments) for lower prices and the response of entrepreneurs trying to gain a larger market share by providing an acceptable product at a lower price. Managed care sneaked up on physicians;

Robert Kuttner, "Must Good HMO's Go Bad? The Commercialization of Prepaid Group Health Care," from *New England Journal of Medicine*, vol. 338, 1558–1563. © 1998 by the Massachusetts Medical Society. Reprinted by permission of the publisher.

by the time they fully grasped the implications, it was a *fait accompli*. Physicians are now caught between patients anxious about the availability and reliability of care and payers demanding further cost control through often perverse financial pressure on doctors.

HMOS: Social or Commercial?

One can distinguish broadly between socially oriented and market-oriented forms of managed care. The socially oriented form realizes efficiencies in three main ways, all rooted in the early nonprofit group plans. First, these plans emphasize prevention and patient education, in addition to treating the sick. This preventive investment, in turn, logically assumes a long-term relationship between the member and the plan.

Second, since there is no monetary incentive to treat patients, the plans pursue cost-effective care. Money saved by reducing unnecessary surgery, excessive inpatient days, preventable illnesses, and so on can be directed toward better prevention and care. Any incentive to undertreat or overtreat is avoided by putting physicians on salary, so that clinical decisions are neutral with respect to income.

Third, the plans carefully monitor what their physicians do in order to educate them about the "best practice" and reduce unjustified variations from it. Integrated plans also encourage communication and effective case management among participating clinicians. Computers facilitate these strategies by allowing case data, screening records, and standard protocols to be disseminated throughout the system of care.

Market-oriented HMOS have some or all of the following additional features. First and foremost they require that participating physicians assume substantial financial risks with respect to the costs of the care they provide. In small doses, income incentives may help remind doctors that resources are limited and may encourage them to provide cost-effective treatment. However, when doctors' earnings are influenced by large financial incentives not to treat patients, the ethical conflict of interest is stark.

Increasingly, individual doctors in such plans are paid on the basis of capitation—a flat fee per member per month. Taken to an extreme, this strategy essentially turns the doctor into an insurance company, often without adequate actuarial spreading of the risk. As a result, there is a close correlation between the treatment the doctor withholds and the money he or she earns. A 1995 survey by the American Medical Association found that 86% of primary care physicians paid on the basis of capitation had no reinsurance, or "stop-loss" protection, to limit the physician's financial exposure.[5]

Other methods of putting doctors' income at risk include withholding a large portion of income and paying bonuses based on the extent to which financial targets are met. In HMOs that pay doctors on a fee-for-service basis, the cost discipline typically entails intensive utilization reviews and, at the extreme, "de-selecting" (firing) doctors who generate above-average costs, both to get rid of the "outliers" and to set an example for others. Other plans make doctors shareholders, so that their income is substantially dependent on controlling expenditures.

Second, primary care physicians are required to serve as gatekeepers. As part of a system of comprehensive, coordinated care, this approach can be constructive. But the gatekeeping role is often counterproductive when coupled with large financial inducements to keep patients from seeing specialists, since specialists are often the appropriate physicians in complex cases. A 1995 survey of 62 independent practice association (IPA) HMOs by the American Society of Internal Medicine found that 88% used a gatekeeping system that required the patient's primary care physician to make all referrals to specialists.[6]

Third, some plans manage costs by carefully selecting the patients they insure. In contrast to the traditional group plans, which welcomed all comers, these plans target employers and industries with relatively young, healthy employees. In the case of individual subscribers, selective marketing is used to attract consumers who are in relatively good health. In the Medicare market, exercise programs may be used less to promote fitness than to attract healthy enrollees. This risk selection approach gives the plan an artificial cost advantage by shifting the costs of treating the sickest people to other plans, which are then seen (wrongly) as high-cost, hence inefficient. HMOs, especially in the Medicare market, can encourage the sickest people to go elsewhere by giving them poor service. A study by Ware and colleagues found that chronically ill elderly and poor patients in three cities had worse clinical outcomes in HMOs than in fee-for-service plans.[7]

Fourth, the sensible imperative to reduce needless variation can translate into simple pressure to reduce utilization per se. An exhaustive 1996 survey of capitation by the Advisory Board Company, a large firm that both provides consultation for and reports on health plans and hospitals, concluded, "To date, capitated systems (principally capitated primary care practices) have achieved savings largely by blocking specialist referrals and hospital admissions altogether."[8]

Many plans now use external vendors for preapproval and utilization review. At some point, there is a plain conflict of interest between the plan's desire to save money and the patient's need for good care. At that point, money is saved not by maximizing quality but by stinting on services, shifting the costs of care to the patient's family or the physician, and sometimes increasing suffering. George Halvorson, chief executive officer of the widely admired Health Partners plan of Minneapolis, draws a useful distinction between "managing care" and merely "managing costs."

Who Is Driving Out Whom?

All these shifts raise an intriguing question. Are the more aggressive forms driving out the more socially conscious forms—or vice versa? This question, in turn, invites several subordinate questions. Has the competitive pressure to cut costs reached a point where socially oriented HMOs embrace practices they once abhorred just to stay in business? Or is the widely touted quality movement preventing a race to the bottom? Alternatively, can self-regulation or government regulation curb unsavory practices?

Is a nonprofit status roughly synonymous with the more ethical brand of HMO? Do the pressures to satisfy shareholders lead to a harsher and more rapacious brand of managed care? Or do they result in better management, giving the for-profit plans a legitimate advantage in the competition for quality and market share? Finally, are many of these questions becoming moot because of the growing emulation of for-profit cost-cutting techniques by nonprofit plans, hence a convergence between ostensibly different kinds of HMO?

Consider a few examples along the spectrum of HMOs.

A Social Ethic

At one end of the spectrum is the Group Health Cooperative of Puget Sound, a consumer cooperative begun in 1945 that remains largely faithful to the traditional model. Group Health still pays doctors a straight salary, with an incentive system that can alter total compensation by only about 2%. Its board is still elected by members of the cooperative, and its medical director is elected by participating doctors. Originally, in line with traditional cooperative principles, Group Health accepted only individual members. In the 1950s, it began signing contracts with large employers and soon became the largest health plan in the Northwest; today it has about 660,000 members.[2]

In response to cost-cutting pressures, which emerged in the 1980s, Group Health made some compromises. It entered into contracts with outside hospitals. The plan has kept its budget for patient care level since 1993, representing a real, inflation-adjusted cut of 23%; this has increased the average doctor's caseload by about 20%. The plan also shifted from pure community rating—charging all members the same premium—to modified community rating based on age, but it departs from the pure form less than its commercial competitors. And in March 1997, to the regret of some traditionalists, the plan negotiated an alliance with Kaiser Permanente, which makes Group Health the Kaiser affiliate in the Northwest. However, Group Health retains operating autonomy and the right to dissolve the affiliation.

What Group Health has not done is to embrace a system of external approvals and denials. "If a doctor orders it, it's covered," according to Dr. Alvin Truscott, until recently Group Health's medical director. Nor has the cooperative made individual doctors financially liable for clinical decisions. Its bonus fund (totaling less than 2% of its $120 million budget for physician compensation) is allocated at the group or clinic level according to three criteria: patient satisfaction; screening, immunization, and other performance goals; and overall budgetary targets. Group Health remains a leader in the type of integrated case management that the entire industry professes to offer.[9]

Kaiser Permanente, Group Health's new big brother, with more than 9 million members, has made more compromises. Although Kaiser still scores high in most rankings and has avoided putting physicians at substantial financial risk, 1997 was its *annus horribilis*. The plan lost $270 million that year because of having overbuilt hospitals in the 1980s and early 1990s. Also in 1997, Kaiser alienated its members and was publicly embarrassed when its underutilized and understaffed hospitals had some disastrous (and widely publicized) clinical outcomes, and then when the plan closed some hospitals to save money. In July, the California Supreme Court held that Kaiser's appeals process was rigged in favor of the plan and ordered a more independent review system. Despite being a nonprofit closely allied with organized labor, Kaiser nonetheless faced bitter strikes by nurses last summer. (The contract settlement, reached in March, included a novel provision empowering nurses to question managerial practices that might compromise the quality of care.)

Unlike Group Health of Puget Sound, Kaiser aims to be a national company. Chief executive officer Dr. David Lawrence said in an interview that in a decade he expects there will be fewer than a dozen national health insurance companies, and he expects Kaiser to be one of them. So although most of its California members still belong to a traditional prepaid group health plan, Kaiser has acquired a widely scattered group of affiliates, many of them network or IPA plans that are a far cry from the original model.

Yet Kaiser continues to score high on both patient satisfaction and more objective indicators. In the Pacific Business group on Health's 1997 rankings, Kaiser, despite its reverses, remained the top-rated California HMO.[10] And notwithstanding competitive pressures, Kaiser has retained adjusted community rating, at least in California, and does not practice risk selection in its marketing. With relatively low disenrollment rates and half a century of experience, Kaiser has perhaps the most comprehensive patient data base of any health plan, which it uses to promote integrated patient care. Since these programs are devised and directed by clinicians, the subculture seems less adversarial than in many commercial HMOs whose primary goal is cost cutting. Lawrence remains a passionate spokesman for the view that nonprofit HMOs are better able to serve patients and preserve the vital doctor-patient relationship. What remains uncertain is whether Kaiser's national expansion will maintain the high standards of its core California plan.

Drifting Away?

Other well-regarded nonprofit plans, such as Harvard Pilgrim Health Care and Tufts Associated Health Plan, two of the leading plans in New England, have moved further away from the traditional HMO model. Tufts, though nominally an HMO in part, is mainly a network. Its 950,000 members select primary care doctors from a list of physicians who may be affiliated with Tufts through a group-practice contract, a hospital-based physician–hospital organization, or a separate contract ("carve-out") in the case of some specialists.

Tufts uses many of the cost-containment methods pioneered by the for-profit HMOs. It pays some doctors on a discounted fee-for-service basis, with incentives that represent about 15% of compensation. The plan also uses capitation to pay some groups of doctors; the groups, in turn, may use capitation to pay their participating doctors or a blend of fee-for-service and incentive payments. According to Dr. Harris Berman, chief executive officer of the Tufts plan, the relevant distinction between plans is not profit status (Tufts has a for-profit subsidiary in New Hampshire) but ownership. "Unlike a shareholder-owned HMO, I can have a bad year or two and not face terrible pressures to reduce care," he said in an interview.

Harvard Pilgrim Health Care has also drifted away from the original Harvard Community Health Plan staff model (which dates back to 1969), largely because of competitive pressure. Of its approximately 1.3 million members in Massachusetts, Rhode Island, New Hampshire, and Maine, only about 300,000 are still in the original plan, which recently changed its name to Harvard Vanguard and shifted from a staff model to a multi-specialty group paid partly on the basis of capitation. The rest of the subscribers are in a broad network of plans that Harvard Pilgrim either purchased or organized. The core HMO membership is slowly shrinking, whereas the network grew last year by 122,000 members.

According to Harvard Pilgrim's medical doctor, Dr. Joseph Dorsey, the fraction of a physician's income that is at risk is typically about 10% in the core Harvard Vanguard plan, which is higher than the fraction at Kaiser and Group Health of Puget Sound but well below that at the more aggressive commercial HMOs. Substantially more compensation may be at risk for doctors in the Harvard Pilgrim network, and some Vanguard executives want to raise the at-risk portion. Harvard Pilgrim also uses a fairly strict gatekeeping system for referrals to most specialists, although members of the Vanguard program may seek care directly from specialists within the network. Like Tufts and most other major nonprofit plans, Harvard Pilgrim continues to have a medical loss ratio (the percentage of premium income spent on care) well above 90%, and the plan scores well on patient satisfaction.

The Market Ethic

At the other end of the spectrum from Group Health of Puget Sound are the entrepreneurial commercial HMOs. As a group, they tend to engage in more aggressive risk selection, use more stringent systems of approval and denial of care, and put a higher fraction of physicians' income at risk.

For example, U.S. Healthcare, the HMO acquired by Aetna, puts roughly half the gross income of its physicians at financial risk. One component of the risk, affecting 10 to 15% of income, is a bonus system that rewards doctors for meeting clinical and marketing goals and achieving a high level of patient satisfaction. A second, larger component rewards or punishes doctors financially on the basis of the clinical costs they incur.

A sample U.S. Healthcare contract sent to participating physicians assumes that a hypothetical Dr. Mahan has 925 patients. His base monthly pay, already adjusted for meeting quality targets, is $7,006. Dr. Mahan can qualify for an additional $3,839 by holding down hospital admissions, emergency room use, and referrals to specialists. Otherwise, he forfeits part or all of the bonus. For example, if his caseload accounts for more than 392 acute care hospital-days per 1,000 enrollees per year, he loses all of a potential $2,063 monthly bonus. To collect the full bonus, he must keep hospital use below 192 days per 1,000. A similar incentive applies to referrals to specialists and emergency room use.[11]

Note that the roughly 50% at-risk figure understates the risk, since it refers to gross income. If, hypothetically, it costs $125,000 to keep the office open, and the doctor normally expects a net income of at least $125,000 on top of that, 50% of gross income (which is $250,000) is really 100% of take-home income at risk.

There is an emerging consensus that for the law of averages to work with payment on the basis of capitation, an individual physician should have at least 250 to 300 enrolled patients.[12] But with "full-risk," or "global," capitation, doctors sometimes accept much smaller numbers of patients on a per-member-per-month contract that makes the doctor financially responsible for most medical costs incurred, including drug and hospital costs, with protection offered only by stop-loss coverage. Capitation is especially problematic when an individual doctor, often a specialist, contracts with a health plan to accept the risk of treating an entire panel of patients, or when the per-member-per-month capitation payment is unrealistically low. Regulations issued December 31, 1996, by the Health Care Financing Administration require plans that put "substantial" physician income at risk, defined as 25% or more, to have stop-loss coverage for 90% of the costs of referrals that exceed the budgeted limit. Such plans are also required to survey members in order to ascertain the quality of care. These rules pertain only to Medicare and Medicaid plans.[13] However, the incentive to deny care is offset only partly by reinsurance or stop-loss coverage, which limits the doctor's financial exposure in catastrophically expensive cases. The financial incentive to withhold or limit care remains pervasive in the great majority of cases.

California-based Pacificare Health Systems, one of the pioneers of capitation, actively encourages large groups of physicians or physician-hospital organizations to accept full risk for all medical events, including inpatient care. Ninety percent of its 2.1 million California enrollees are in a globally capitated plan. The groups, in turn, have a wide range of incentive-payment systems for their participating doctors. Pacificare has no contracts with individual physicians.

Oxford Health Plans, another variant of the for-profit HMO, pursued market share by offering patients generous benefits and paying most affiliated doctors on a fee-for-service basis—a relatively light-handed form of managed care. The company advertised aggressively, targeting a relatively young, affluent population in the hope that favorable selection would offset the liberal benefits and payments to physicians. The company grew from under 100,000 subscribers in 1992 to 2 million subscribers in late 1997.[14]

For a time, Oxford was the darling of Wall Street. Its chief executive officer, Stephen Wiggins, was an apostle of shareholder-owned HMOs, who regularly denounced nonprofit plans as inefficient tax evaders. Wiggins's formula seemed too good to be true, and it was. Despite its demographic targeting, Oxford became known as a good plan to have if you had a costly, chronic condition. According to Susan Dooha of the Gay Men's Health Crisis in New York, Oxford—to the plan's chagrin—was well regarded by people at risk of contracting AIDS. By the third quarter of 1997, the company was reporting a medical loss ratio of nearly 100% and had to delay its payments to doctors. The problem was blamed on computer foul-ups, but in part it reflected an overly sanguine business strategy. Before the stock crashed, Wiggins personally exercised some $27.3 million in stock options.

Health Partners, based in Minneapolis, is an example of a nonprofit plan that uses market-like disciplines in a system that retains a strong social commitment and good checks and balances. The plan, which serves about 800,000 subscribers, is the result of a merger of five nonprofit organizations plus a teaching hospital; it includes staff model HMOs, network HMOs, and contracts with multispecialty groups. Like Group Health of Puget Sound, Health Partners is organized as a cooperative. It disseminates information to subscribers on the performance of the several units in the system, which in effect compete with each other for patients. The plan even puts its comparative performance data on the Internet (http://www.consumerchoice.com), and usage is running at more than 50,000 contacts ("hits") per month. Like the other, more socially minded HMOs, Health Partners limits the portion of a physician's income at risk to about 5%. Minnesota is the only remaining state that requires HMOs to be non-profit, and Health Partners lobbies hard to keep it that way.

A Partial Convergence

One of the original promises of prepaid group health was to improve coordination of services. It is ironic, then, that despite a lot of talk about "virtual staff models," many nominal HMOs today are actually far-flung assortments of doctors with strict utilization controls or financial incentives but little ongoing interaction, much less a common approach to practice. For-profit plans are leading this trend, but some nonprofit plans are following suit because of competitive pressures.

Managed care under market auspices has thus produced a double paradox. The more patients chafe under the constraints of utilization controls, the more they demand a choice of doctors—not realizing that the various doctors affiliated with a plan have similar or identical financial incentives to constrain costs. And the more plans try to offer a choice, the further they stray from the systemwide integration, prevention, and case management that are the supposed advantages of HMOs. Some of the most entrepreneurial HMOs, such as Pacificare and Oxford, pride themselves on no longer requiring that referrals to specialists be made by primary care doctors; they count instead on financial incentives for participating specialists to hold down costs. A Health Care Advisory Board report quotes an unnamed chief executive officer of a health plan as saying, "If you're going to offer consumers more choice, you can't hold medical groups responsible for the care they don't manage."[15]

The shift away from staff-model HMOs may also be attractive to plan executives because it reduces counterpressure by physicians. It is difficult for doctors in a loose network of practices, linked only by contracts, to resist clinical intrusions in a deliberate and concerted manner. Plans that are still group- or staff-model HMOs, such as Kaiser Permanente's California plan, must continually negotiate with their doctors about the clinical terms of managed care. In contrast, a physician who contracts with 5 or 10 HMO networks, each with particular strategies and protocols, is likely to have little influence over the terms and may see the required reports, profiles, clinical guidelines, and meetings not as emblems of teamwork but as unnecessary intrusions and paperwork. It is unclear whether the integration and case-management benefits of true HMOs can be achieved in loose networks.[16,17]

Well-managed and poorly managed HMOs can be found in both ownership categories. Despite the superior management often attributed to for-profit ownership, many commercial HMOs have suffered from far greater volatility (because of mergers, acquisitions, divestments, periodic reversals of business strategy, and competition for market share) as well as higher rates of disenrollment on the part of both patients and physicians. The nonprofit HMOs include relatively well-managed plans such as Group Health of Puget Sound, Tufts, and Harvard Pilgrim, which have sound business plans and strong systems of financial and clinical accountability. But other nonprofit HMOs, such as the Health Insurance Plan of Greater New York and several Blue Cross–Blue Shield plans, are notorious for poor management.

Are Nonprofit Plans Better?

Despite the partial convergence of for-profit and nonprofit plans, the nonprofit plans as a group tend to score better on many objective indicators and in surveys of consumers. A December 1997 study of all Medicare HMOs, which relied on data from the Health Care Financing Administration, used disenrollment as a rough proxy for consumer satisfaction. Of the 10 plans with the lowest disenrollment rates (less than 6% on average), 9 were nonprofit plans. Of the 10 plans with the highest turnover (about 50% on average), 7 were for-profit plans.[18] In Consumers Union's 1996 consumer-satisfaction survey of HMOs, the 11 top-ranked HMOs were nonprofit plans, and 12 of the 13 bottom-ranked HMOs were for-profit plans.[19] *U.S. News and World Report*'s 1997 survey, which used data from the National Committee for Quality Assurance, gave HMOs a composite score based on such factors as prevention, physician and member turnover and satisfaction, access to care, and accreditation. Of the 37 top-scoring HMOs, 33 were nonprofit plans.[20] Comparisons of medical loss ratios generally show that nonprofit plans are more efficient. They characteristically spend more than 90 cents of the premium dollar on health care, whereas expenditures by the better commercial HMOs tend to be closer to 80 cents on the dollar, and expenditures by the most aggressive HMOs are in the range of 70 or even 60 cents on the dollar.

In sum, although nonprofit status seems to be conducive to a less harsh form of managed care, it is no guarantee. The relentless pressure to cut costs will undoubtedly continue. The key question is whether counterpressures will provide adequate checks and balances. In principle, counterpressures can be generated by informed consumers with a meaningful choice of competing plans, professional ethics, the quality movement, industry self-regulation, and the growing bipartisan drive for government regulation.

Notes

1   Starr P. *The social transformation of American medicine.* New York: Basic Books, 1982.
2   Crowley W. *To serve the greatest number.* Seattle: University of Washington Press, 1996.
3   *Market facts, February 1998.* Menlo Park, Calif.: Henry J. Kaiser Family Foundation, 1998.
4   Nelson H. *Nonprofit and for-profit HMOs: converging practices but different goals?* New York: Milbank Memorial Fund, 1997:1.
5   Simon CJ, Emmons DW. Physician earnings at risk: an examination of capitated contracts. *Health Aff* (Millwood) 1997; 16(3):120–6.
6   Patient access to internist-subspecialists in gatekeeper health plans. Washington, D.C.: *American Society of Internal Medicine,* August 1995: 6.
7   Ware JE Jr, Bayliss MS, Rogers WH, Kosinski M, Tarlov AR. Differences in 4-year health outcomes for elderly and poor, chronically ill patients treated in HMO and fee-for-service systems: results from the Medical Outcomes Study. *JAMA* 1996; 276:1039–47.
8   *Capitation strategy.* Washington, D.C.: Advisory Board, 1996: 171.
9   Thompson RS. What have HMOs learned about clinical prevention services? An examination of the experience at Group Health Cooperative of Puget Sound. *Milbank Q* 1996; 74(4):469–509.
10 *Consumer satisfaction with HMOs.* San Francisco: Pacific Business Group on Health, 1997.
11 *Quality care compensation system: monthly sample reporting package.* Blue Bell, Pa.: Aetna U.S. Healthcare, 1997.
12 *Assuring appropriate patient care under capitation arrangements.* Washington, D.C.: American Society of Internal Medicine, August 1995.
13 *Requirements for physician incentive plans.* No. 42CFR417.479. Rev. ed. Washington, D.C.: Health Care Financing Administration, October 1, 1997.
14 *Report to the Securities and Exchange Commission, Form 10-Q.* Oxford Health Plans, September 30, 1997.
15 *Future revenues: sustainable growth strategies for America's health systems.* Washington, D.C.: Health Care Advisory Board, 1997:15.
16 Luft HS, Greenlick MR. The contribution of group- and staff-model HMOs to American medicine. *Milbank Q* 1996; 74(4):445–67.
17 Gold MR, Hurley R, Lake T, Ensor T, Berenson R. A national survey of the arrangement managed-care plans make with physicians. *N Engl J Med* 1995; 333:1678–83.
18 *Comparing Medicare HMOs: do they keep their members?* Washington, D.C.: Families USA, 1997.
19 *Consumer Reports,* August 1996:40–1.
20 The HMO honor roll. *U.S. News & World Report.* October 23, 1997:62.

Defending My Life
Geov Parrish

I nearly died.

Several times.

That I am alive to write such words—any words—explains my nearly unfathomable loyalty to the women and men of the University of Washington Medical Center's organ transplant program. They saved my life, and have since kept me alive and in (mostly) relatively good health. Their handiwork is close to my heart.

About 10 inches south.

My story is important to me, but it's nearly routine for practitioners of advanced high-tech medicine who perform these procedures that extend lives and often offer a good quality of life to those saved. But: they're frighteningly expensive; they are as seemingly random (in a perverse way) as the death penalty in selecting who gets the chance to live; and they operate independently of the resource needs of simpler, preventive public health programs that, if applied around the world, could save millions of lives each year.

My involvement began just over 10 years ago, when a nephrologist (kidney specialist) with the bedside manner of a gargoyle sat at her desk, eyes fixed absently on some point high on the opposite wall, and casually told me that I was likely to be dead in a year or two or three. This same reputable but inaccessible doctor proceeded to ignore me over the next two years, damn near ensuring the accuracy of her prediction. All the while, my condition steadily worsened, and my insurance company balked over the necessity and expense of a simultaneous transplant of two organs: a kidney and a pancreas. Due to a congressional oddity, Medicare covers kidney transplants, but at the time it wouldn't cover the pancreas—and neither would my insurers, because they considered the procedure "experimental." I needed both organs to live.

In September 1993, I lapsed briefly into a coma and then began dialysis treatments for my failed kidneys. For five hours a day, three days a week, a needle the size of a pencil transported my blood through an artificial kidney machine, filtering out the impurities.

Some people's bodies cope well with dialysis; as with most Type I diabetics, mine did not. I wound up with seven or eight surgeries to repair and/or unclot the artificial blood vessel in my right arm used for the dialysis procedure. After a month, increasingly erratic blood sugars put me in the hospital again. I could no longer work at my part-time job as a community activist. On November 12, I started convulsing while dancing at a party and was out of it again for a couple of days. Two weeks later, my then wife Kiyoko found me passed out in the shower, and she and a group of friends I will never forget (Vivien, Gavin, Carolyn, Ellen, Scott, Lisa, and Lance, among others) stood watch as I lay in a coma for several days.

Once I emerged from the medication-induced hallucinogenic hell that followed, we changed doctors, and UWMC got serious about taking the only course of action likely to work. With better medical care, my condition was poor but more stable. The insurance company finally, reluctantly, agreed to save my life. In June, I got a pager, for use when compatible organs were found. Every few weeks, someone would call a wrong number, and I'd damn near have a heart attack. Then, on the evening of December 16, 1994, the pager went off for real. In only six months, they'd found a "match," from an 18-year-old man (bless him) killed in an auto accident in Portland. It was four months before my insurance would expire due to Kiyoko's having been laid off. I had just turned 35.

The 10-hour surgery the next morning proved successful. It also represented a lifelong commitment on my behalf by UWMC's doctors. Like the staff at most transplant programs, they don't like to see their patients die after so much time and effort, and so, even though I can't really afford it, they continue to be aggressive in my care. In six years, I've had a stroke, a possible rejection episode, two bouts with double pneumonia, a nasty (and potentially life-threatening) cryptococcal fungal infection, and taken over $100,000 in immunosuppressant drugs. That's pretty good; I know K-P patients who've had a much rougher go. Not everyone lives. For the decade, I've resulted in around a million dollars in health care expenses billed to insurance. I am the insurance industry's worst nightmare. I lived.

By acting to save myself, I took advantage of a global health care system that, in the name of profitability, intentionally fails far more people than it saves. How many more people would now be alive if the million dollars spent on one person—me—had instead been spent on medical vouchers in Lake City? Or vaccines in Chad, or water filters in Tanzania, or a health clinic on a Lakota reservation? Dozens? Hundreds? Thousands? Each year, that question becomes more urgent, as thousands of beneficiaries of new treatments—transplants, protease inhibitors, fancy new tests—not only live when we wouldn't have 20 or even 5 years ago, but proceed to require expensive health care treatments for as long as we remain alive.

Not everybody gets that chance. Money, of course, matters, beginning with whether someone has enough regular access to health care to have been diagnosed in time for procedures like mine to work. It also takes a certain kind of assertiveness to navigate the byzantine, often dehumanizing world of specialized health care.

From the doctor's side, whether someone can take advantage of high-end medicine depends on a number of factors. Dr. Christopher Marsh, associate director of UWMC's Division of Transplantation, ticks off the eligibility requirements for a liver, kidney, or pancreas transplant: "Getting referred by primary care; being medically suitable—that is, being compliant, not having severe co-morbid conditions; having psychosocial support; not having mental illness—though it doesn't preclude you if you're under control. We look at a patient's financial status, but in actuality we can get through the transplant and surgery financially." Marsh says that insurance companies and HMOs can be more of a financial barrier than the hospital: "They can be a substantial gatekeeper and not refer patients, or refer them too late, or send them to a center that is cheaper but doesn't give the best results, or not refer them back to long-term care."

Candidates must be clean of substance abuse, a particular issue for liver patients who've destroyed their health through years of alcohol abuse; at UWMC, says one administrator, "If there's any kind of substance abuse, they have to go through a formal rehab program. The patient can't just say, well, I quit. . . . You have to look at it as giving people a chance." And then matching organs have to be found. According to Marsh, the average wait time is now two years for a pancreas or liver.

In 1994, I met all the medical conditions, and my organs showed up in six months. Were I in the same situation now, I would wait much longer for matching organs, which is a severe medical risk, but insurance coverage would not be as critical of an issue. Medicare covers all treatment of kidney disease—including, as of about three years ago, the costs of kidney-pancreas transplants as well.

Our national health care system is a pyramid of such legislative flukes. Dr. Christopher Blagg, director emeritus of the Northwest Kidney Foundation, the area's oldest and largest dialysis provider, says that over 30 years ago, "the Senate decided, over a weekend almost, to fund dialysis treatment . . . they honestly didn't know what it was going to cost." Kidney transplants were subsequently covered, and when joint kidney-pancreas transplants came along, it was discovered that they, too, were cheaper than a lifetime of dialysis.

Dr. Kim Muczynski, my current nephrologist and the director of UWMC's renal clinic, says that 11 of Washington state's insurers now enforce a one-year wait for kidney and kidney-pancreas transplants. The hope is that patients will be forced on to dialysis, in which case Medicare, rather than the insurance company, picks up the cost of the transplant.

The dilemma I faced over coverage for a new, or even relatively new, procedure is common. Hugh Straley, an oncologist who is Group Health Cooperative's associate medical director, helps decide whether Group Health will pay for an experimental procedure. "In most cases," Straley says, "most insurers do not cover experimental treatment."

"We're looking for the grade of evidence: high grade (rigorous randomized controlled trial), or low grade (description of small group of patients), or clinical opinion. What we are really looking for is high-grade evidence. That doesn't mean that there isn't benefit otherwise, just that there isn't evidence; we might approve it anyway. We also assess the impact on the system, the cost to the system, and community standards; we seek input from relevant specialists as well. In most cases, the decisions are relatively easy to make. In other cases, the decisions are much more difficult. The evidence is marginal; the benefits are marginal. We really have to weigh whether this is an appropriate benefit for a small group of people. If the evidence is that it is life-saving, we'll cover it."

However, the evidence—and the definition of "life-saving"—is in the eye of the beholder. A terminally ill patient is likely to want alternatives, regardless of the rigorousness of the evidence. And so, three years ago, Straley and Group Health found themselves in the middle of a conflict. Teri Lafnitzegger, a 37-year-old Kitsap County housewife suffering from an aggressive, deadly brain tumor, wanted to go to North Carolina to try an experimental therapy offered at Duke University.

Group Health Cooperative physicians gave her a few months to live and would not pay for her care at Duke. Media coverage and a firestorm of public sympathy helped convince Group Health to relent. At an emotional public forum in February 1999, in which Lafnitzegger confronted Straley and Group Health officials, she pointed to her presence at the forum as evidence that the therapy worked and was worth paying for.

Seven months later, Teri passed away. She got to see her youngest child enter kindergarten. Both she and her husband, Eric, thought the Duke therapy gave her several extra months of life. Today, Eric still thinks the Duke treatment was the right thing to do.

And Straley has doubts. He says that the procedure they tried "still hasn't panned out. It's still of marginal value. . . . From her and her family's point of view, it's worth it . . . but for a hundred patients with brain tumors who have a shortened life expectancy, is it worth it to spend $50,000—$100,000 for each patient to get one or several months of additional survival for a small percentage of them? That is one of the most difficult things we can do. We generally say that it's not, that the scarce resource can be better applied to the larger population."

While insurance companies, in denying high-cost treatments, can claim that they are trying to ensure lower-cost health care reimbursement for more people, the big transnational corporations that dominate the pharmaceutical industry have no such excuses. Drugs like cyclosporin are lifesavers; the greed of their manufacturers can be a major barrier to equitable health care. For someone in the United States, it's a struggle; for someone in the Third World with AIDS, cancer, or a transplant, it's a death sentence. It's been well publicized, for example, that some of these companies have fought mightily—with U.S. government support—to prevent inexpensive generic anti-AIDS drugs from being distributed in the Third World.

But all forms of health care are maldistributed. Muczynski notes that kidney transplants—common for decades in this country—are performed in the Third World only with a living donor, and patients suffering from kidney failure aren't given dialysis unless a transplant is lined up. For patients who can afford it, however, Third World transplants are actually much cheaper. Muczynski knows of a Filipino patient who went back to his country and, for $5,000, had a kidney transplant that would have cost him $33,000 here. The United States, of course, has better care and monitoring, but of the enormous price gap, she shrugs, "It's just the way we do things." In fact, doctors and hospitals lose money on some types of transplants; the problem lies with the stunning variety of expenses we build in.

Profit is one of those expenses, and at times the impact is immediate. Last winter, the United States suffered a shortage of flu vaccines, in large part because a manufacturer chose to redirect two of its factories to produce a more profitable drug. According to one industry observer who didn't want to be named, "obscene drug company profits cost lives in the U.S. If there's a 10% margin for a heart attack drug instead of 50%, it won't be made. A couple of companies have stopped making flu vaccine. Others aren't making enough, because their factories switched over to more profitable drugs. Factories making these basic drugs are now making Viagra instead."

The biggest financial problem, for me and for most transplant patients, comes well after the survey. Jeff Harder, a UWMC social worker who helps patients find financial resources, says, "In eight years I don't remember ever turning down a patient for the transplant itself because of finances, but there's a big variety in how insurance companies cover prescription drugs." Medicare covers prescription drug costs for only three years post-transplant; after that, most of us are on our own, no matter how disabled.

Six years out from my successful transplants, I go through 42 pills, two oral solutions, and two patches every day. That includes the immunosuppressant drugs that, by preventing organ rejection, keep me alive. Every transplant patient, everywhere in the world, takes these drugs for the rest of their lives. Cyclosporin, which revolutionized transplant surgery in 1984, isn't costly to make and long ago repaid its developmental and marketing costs. Yet because one company holds the international patent, the manufacturer is able to gouge. I'm billed $1,037.73 a month for the form of cyclosporin I take. For me, it means that I'm kept alive by my access to insurance, because uninsured, my drug bill is more than my monthly income. And insurance companies, in Washington state, are desperate to jettison the chronically ill, a right which the state legislature gave them last year. Neither the state nor federal programs like Medicare have comprehensive strategies for addressing the health care costs of the growing population of chronically ill.

As governments cut spending not directly related to making business happy, public health provisions for things like food and water safety lose funding ground. Debbie Ward, a former board chair of Group Health also involved in the Lafnitzegger case, points out, "The things that make the biggest difference to the public's health aren't individual services. They're public health services like water safety. Of the things that make a huge difference to public health, first we have these deeply undervalued public health issues. Then, well, it probably turns out to be things like income, and job safety, and neighborhood safety. . . . The disproportionate amount of money that's spent on . . . surgical interventions that make small differences, medical interventions that make small differences, aren't as important as these things."

My case exemplifies the point about public health. My kidney disease was a complication of Type I diabetes—which came from pancreatic failure that occurred when I contracted a viral infection from bad drinking water. If the drinking water in Eastland, Texas, hadn't been infected one day in August 1977, I probably wouldn't have racked up a million dollars in health care costs in the 1990s.

One of the more benevolent reasons insurance companies have been reluctant to pay for high-cost treatments, beyond the cost itself, is that it saves more lives to spend the same amount of money on preventive procedures instead. Preventive medicine has historically suffered in America because it's not as profitable in the short term as expensive specialties and high-tech responses to acute illness. Slowly, that's changing; "wellness" as a term didn't exist 20 years ago. Now insurance companies and HMOs emphasize prevention.

Muczynski is optimistic on this front: "We are thinking now about how to prevent original disease. As transplants are evolving, so are newer therapies and measures to promote awareness early on." Straley concurs: "Primary prevention has always been seen just in terms of public health, but now we're looking at moving to other means of extending life—management of risk factors such as smoking, moderation of alcohol use, exercise, management of nutrition. These interventions translate into longer and better lives."

But the money-driven commitment to wellness has a nasty edge. Illness is expensive. Insurance companies and HMOs prefer "well" patients. And they prefer them to the point where the chronically ill cannot afford, or even obtain, insurance or adequate health care. As baby boomers age, cancer rates soar, and the number of uninsured Americans approaches 50 million, that gatekeeping has become a major crisis. Access to fancy treatments is only a small part of the problem. Straley sees the crisis coming: "When there are 45 million people not getting primary care, that's not a wise public health investment for the U.S. to make."

For me, high-tech medicine has had a wonderful payoff. Not only have I had precious extra years with family and friends, but I'm still alive to agitate for more humane political policies and to make Mark Sidran and Paul Schell's lives less comfortable. That, surely, is worth a large public investment.

But what about the liver transplantee who reverts to alcohol abuse? Should his life not have been saved? What about people like Teri Lafnitzegger, who despite a brave and spirited battle, only got an extra six months? Should we all have been passed over in favor of a more equitable allocation of health resources? How many families of people who died at least in part because of inadequate access to basic health care could trade places with my family?

In 10 years of navigating Seattle's health care facilities, I have met countless health care providers who are agonized because they can't practice medicine appropriately and their patients suffer or even die. The American system is the most technologically advanced, but also by far the most expensive, one of the least efficient, and one of the most economically segregated in the world. Under our current public policies, there's not enough money available to save the lives of everyone whose life could be extended or saved—even in the wealthy United States, let alone the rest of the world.

Usually, the choices are not dramatic, and happen over years on the basis of geography and class and lifestyle and quirks like the federal support for kidney patients. But sometimes, the decision makers have names and desks. Doctors, hospitals, HMOs, drug companies, and especially insurance companies trade in these questions every day. Absent any focused public policy, they're making the calls. Increasingly, in a for-profit health care system, money is driving the decisions.

My original insurance company stalled for three years, claiming that a kidney-pancreas procedure was experimental. Their recalcitrance, while I went through successive comas, nearly killed me. Had I died, they would have saved a lot of money. Had I been wealthy enough to pay for the procedure myself, my life would not have been so endangered.

I'm still not wealthy. It's been nearly a decade since I last worked full time, and while I'm ecstatic to be alive, some days are a lot worse than others. I'm currently self-employed and pay out of my paltry income for my own individual insurance, with additional out-of-pocket medical expenses that leave me with very little to live on and no savings. According to Dr. Muczynski and others, my six-year-old nonnative organs have a finite life span of—under good conditions—roughly 10 years (pancreas) and

15–20 (kidneys). If they're right, in a few short years I'll be battling the same complications and downward spiral that led to my grave illness and original transplants.

At that point, absent my winning the Lotto, my life will again be in the hands of gatekeepers. This time, they won't be concerned about whether the treatment works—it's now well established—but they might be looking at new "experimental" treatments or drugs. If not, they'll wonder whether a second round of transplantation, in a world of scarce organs, should take priority over someone who needs it for the first time. And they'll especially worry about money, and the fact that I've already consumed so much of it.

That, really, is the basic question: Do we, as a society, value the right to make more money over the lives of our neighbors? In the wealthiest society in the history of the world, amidst tax cuts for the wealthy and gazillion-dollar weapon boondoggles, how many lives could we save? Which ones? Do I have a right to demand more? Do I have a right to live?

I think I do. But it's not my decision.

Business vs. Medical Ethics:
Conflicting Standards for Managed Care
Wendy K. Mariner

The increased competition for a share of the market of insured patients, which arose in the wake of failed comprehensive health care reform, has provoked questions about what, if any, standards will govern new "competitive" health care organizations.[1] Managed care arrangements, which typically shift to providers and patients some or all of the financial risk for patient care,[2] are of special concern because they can create incentives to withhold beneficial care from patients.[3] Of course, fee-for-service (FFS) medical practice creates incentives to provide unnecessary services, and managed care can avoid that type of harm.[4] Still, as Edmund Pellegrino has noted, "managed care, by its nature, places the good of the patient into conflict with . . . (1) the good of all the other patients served by the plan; (2) the good of the plan and the organization, themselves . . .; and (3) the self-interest of the physician."[5]

These potential conflicts have sparked a small flurry of articles and conferences that examine the "ethics" of managed care.[6] Participants in this discussion recognize the benefits of managed care, including its focus on disease prevention and health promotion (long overdue in American medical practice), its coordination of services based on the totality of a patient's health needs (rather than on isolated responses to specific symptoms), and its ability to hold down premiums. Yet financial incentives to limit services may undermine managed care's ability to achieve such benefits.

Carolyn Clancy and Howard Brody distinguish good managed care organizations (MCOs), which they call "Jekyll care," from "bad" organizations or "Hyde care."[7] In their view, Jekyll organizations typically are

Wendy K. Mariner, "Business vs. Medical Ethics: Conflicting Standards for Managed Care," from *Journal of Law, Medicine, and Ethics*, vol. 23, 236–246. © 1995 by the American Society of Law, Medicine, and Ethics. Reprinted by permission of the publisher.

well-established, nonprofit health maintenance organizations (HMOS), like Group Health Cooperative of Puget Sound and Kaiser-Permanente Foundation, that encourage coordinated care, including preventive services, in long-term personal relationships between patients and primary care providers. They find bad managed care most often in the newer, investor-owned, for-profit entities operated by insurance companies and managers.[8] With little or no experience in health care delivery, such organizations may focus on cutting costs and on ensuring an adequate return on investment to their shareholders.

The idea that some managed care is good and some bad suggests that some socially accepted standard can be defined against which to judge individual plans. But we have no such standard yet. Indeed, disagreement persists over whether any standard is even necessary. Among those who advocate particular standards, there is implicit disagreement on whether the standard should be based on principles of economics, policy, or ethics; and if ethical principles apply, whether they should be medical ethics or business ethics.

This essay explores the difficulty of adopting ethical standards for MCOS. First, it is not clear what counts as an ethical standard for an organization. The ideals of quality and efficiency are desirable goals but do not describe how they ought to be achieved. The ethical principles that promote free and fair competition are quite different from the ethical principles that preserve the integrity of the physician-patient relationship and specifically those that protect patient welfare, and these principles can lead to quite different outcomes. MCOS were created to achieve economic objectives that may be fundamentally incompatible with traditional principles of medical ethics. Moreover, in today's open-ended health care system, it is questionable whether American economic institutions are susceptible to purely moral suasion. Thus, even if it is possible to agree that certain ethical principles ought to apply to managed care, the market may make it impossible to live fully by those principles.

Finally, it is important not to mistake ethical managed care for an ethical national health care system. Good MCOS may be able to provide efficient, high quality care; but, in the long run, they are not likely to be able to do so and simultaneously cut costs and promote equitable access to care. If the analysis presented here is correct, then we have a choice: either abandon the goal of universal access to health care, or regulate the health care system by eliminating those marketplace standards that conflict with equitable access to care.

Ethical principles are sometimes conflated with economic and political goals. When the Clinton administration's task force was developing the Health Security Act, it invited a group of ethicists to propose principles for the plan. The group's list of 14 principles was reduced to the following 6 for presentation to the public: security, savings, choice, quality, responsibility, and simplicity.[9] These may be laudable goals for health care reform, but, with the possible exception of choice and responsibility, they are not ethical principles.

The current growth of MCOs is encouraged as an alternative to comprehensive health care reform.[10] The Clinton administration's proposal provoked successful opposition from groups who argued that additional government intervention was not needed in the health insurance market because increased competition could achieve the goals of controlling costs and providing good quality care.[11] (They did not claim that competition could achieve universal access to care.) Were care "managed" properly, it could maintain quality and lower costs (or at least limit cost increases). Thus, the goals of managed care came to be seen as the efficient use of health care resources (or controlling costs) to provide quality care.[12] The most politically appealing argument was cost control; and managed care is advocated first and foremost as a cost control mechanism by those who oppose additional government intervention in health care financing.[13]

Today, health insurers only have a limited number of ways to save money: use resources efficiently; pay providers less; shift the risk of loss to providers; exclude costly patients from coverage; reduce covered benefits; limit services and deny treatment claims; and increase deductibles and copayments. It is certainly possible to increase efficiency, and avoid waste and duplication of services, in administering and delivering health care.[14] Still, many knowledgeable commentators believe that, in the long run, efficiency alone will not reduce costs enough to avoid limiting the amount of beneficial services needed by patients,[15] especially where the patient population includes an increasing number of older, sicker people.

The remaining cost control methods are likely to result in reducing services available to patients or increasing patients' out-of-pocket expenditures. For example, insurers can reduce their own costs by lowering the amount they pay providers—especially hospitals and physicians—to care for patients, either by obtaining fee discounts, or by paying providers on a capitated basis (a fixed fee per subscriber) in whole or in part, so that the provider bears the risk of financial loss if the costs of care exceed the capitation fee.[16] Managed care plans may use practice guidelines, quality control committees, and financial rewards and penalties to influence physicians' treatment decisions.[17] Plans may also require patient care to be screened by primary care gatekeepers and employ or contract only with physicians who practice in a cost-saving manner and adhere to the plan's efficient treatment methods.

Historically, most insurers avoided large or unpredictable expenses by refusing to insure patients who were at risk of needing expensive services.[18] The practice of "cherry-picking," or insuring only healthy patients who are unlikely to get sick, is still an effective cost control device.[19] Plans can also encourage patients who require expensive services to leave the plan and join another, by, for example, providing poor or inconvenient service, refusing desired care, or not responding to complaints.[20]

Health plans can limit their expenses by reducing the number and type of medical benefits covered by the plan. Where services are not expressly excluded from the contract, insurers may deny coverage on the grounds that they are not medically necessary, for example.[21] Finally, increased deductibles and copayments shift to patients a larger proportion of the cost of their care, although their contribution to insurer cost savings may be minimal.

The goals of efficiency and quality care are desirable programmatic goals for health plans, but they do not specify ethical standards for their achievement. They may also conflict with one another. Efficiency is unlikely to control costs enough to avoid hard decisions about limitations on care. Defining and measuring quality of care remains problematic.[22] In such circumstances, ethical standards to guide MCOs' actions appear especially needed.

Differences in Medical Ethics and Business Ethics

Can and should ethical standards apply to MCOs? The answer to such a question depends on what counts as an ethical standard. Traditional principles of medical ethics that govern the physician-patient relationship certainly have a role to play in the delivery of medical care, whether it is done in private FFS practice or in integrated service networks.[23] MCOs, however, do more than deliver medical care. They combine insurance, management, and care delivery. It may be argued that the organization itself does not deliver medical care: its physicians and nurses do. The organization is an economic entity, often a corporation—a legal fiction, not a person in a profession with a history of professional ethics. Thus, the ethical principles that have traditionally been thought to apply to health care practitioners do not easily fit MCOs.

Susan Wolf has rightly distinguished between physician's ethics and organizational ethics, arguing for the development of ethical standards for health care organizations.[24] That task faces several obstacles. First, it is debatable whether organizations are moral entities or capable of having ethics at all.[25] Wolf argues that health care organizations qualify as moral agents because they "specify levels of management and care delivery, formulate rules and policies, and consider moral reasons." Of course, most, if not all organizations (including Microsoft and R. J. Reynolds) formulate rules and policies and consider moral reasons for their actions. The fact that corporations make decisions based on moral reasoning does not mean that they must. These two criteria alone do not suffice to describe an institutional moral agent.

What distinguishes health care organizations from other (commercial and nonprofit) enterprises is the fact that they are in the business of delivering health care (Wolf's first factor). Moreover, that health care is actually provided by individual professionals who do have ethical obligations. MCOs perform both medical and business functions, taking actions to provide or withhold care that touch the traditional sphere of medical ethics, and, at the same time, acting like ordinary business enterprises with no moral obligations or, at least, obligations that have little to do with traditional medical ethics. This functional duality gives health care organizations a foot in both the medical and the business camps.

However, it is not necessary to confer moral agency on organizations in order to hold them to ethical standards of conduct. Whether or not organizations are moral entities or have moral rights or duties, their actions can be judged by moral standards and either praised or condemned.[26] Organizations can voluntarily create institutional structures and policies that require or encourage ethical behavior on the part of their personnel. Moreover, ethical standards of conduct can be legally imposed where it is socially desirable to achieve important goals.[27] The more difficult tasks will be developing the content of standards that take into account the dual business and medical functions of MCOs and ensuring that organizations can adhere to such standards in an increasingly competitive environment.

The types of standards that have been proposed for managed care entities tend to reflect different conceptions of the organization—either its medical functions or its business functions, but not both. Those who seek ethical standards to ensure the delivery of high quality care appear to conceive of the organization as an entity that has or should have moral obligations because of its medical care functions.[28] The standards they propose focus on preserving physicians' traditional (or updated) ethical commitment to patient welfare despite financial and management controls designed to restrict the cost of care. Others appear to conceive of the organization as a purely economic enterprise, a business with no moral obligations to patients.[29] The standards they discuss are not ethical principles, but management goals, such as economic efficiency, product quality, information dissemination, and fair competition. A consensus on standards is unlikely unless these conflicting views are reconciled.

Problems with Business Ethics

Business ethics in the United States deal with the ethical conduct of business in a competitive marketplace.[30] The ethical principles governing business are designed to promote fair competition. These include honesty, truthfulness, and keeping promises. More specific principles give content to these general principles. For example, business people should avoid disseminating information that is false or misleading and avoid exploiting relationships for personal gain.

Fair competition assumes some measure of equality among those who do business, and seeks to assure conditions in which people are free to make voluntary choices to buy or sell goods or services. Medical ethics, in contrast, assumes significant inequality in knowledge and skill between physicians and patients. For this reason, physicians have been found to have a type of fiduciary obligation to their patients. Business organizations do not have fiduciary obligations to their customers. Their fiduciary obligations are to their shareholders, in the case of investor-owned, for-profit enterprises,[31] or to the state, in the case of nonprofit organizations. Investor-owned businesses are expected to preserve their assets to accomplish the organization's business purpose and to provide a financial return to investors. Nonprofit organizations must also use their resources to accomplish a stated noncommercial purpose.

MCOs face difficulties when achievement of their mission to provide medical care conflicts with their obligation to preserve their assets. This is especially true in the case of for-profit MCOs, which may be under pressure to maintain stock prices and to pay dividends. Some commercial

organizations have attempted to adopt socially responsible corporate policies, such as producing or using products that do not harm the environment. Often, such products are both popular and profitable, so that the
company can satisfy both its customers and its shareholders. Similarly,
many MCOs hope that patient satisfaction will attract new subscribers
and, hence, sufficient revenues to yield a satisfactory return to investors.
Investors or shareholders of an MCO, however, are rarely the same people
as those enrolled in the health plan. If an MCO's financial goals conflict
with its service methods, little in the field of business ethics argues for
giving subscribers priority.

Stanley Reiser offers the following values to guide health care institutions: humaneness, reciprocal benefit, trust, fairness, dignity, gratitude,
service, and stewardship.[32] Apart from fairness, such values are not generally included in discussions of American business values as freedom (to
buy and sell), profit, fairness (including honesty and truthfulness), equal
opportunity, and pragmatism or efficiency.[33] Some of Reiser's values may
be incompatible with achieving the MCO's financial goals. For example,
his concept of reciprocal benefit restrains institutions from actions that
harm some to benefit others. MCOs, however, may have to allocate their
resources in ways that explicitly harm some patients or providers to benefit others, so to use resources efficiently to provide the most services to
an entire enrollee population. The notion of service, or the obligation
to use one's talents to benefit others rather than to expect rewards for
labor, is similarly problematic. MCOs typically assume the opposite; they
frequently use financial rewards and penalties to influence physician behavior, for example. In addition, humaneness, which encompasses compassion for people, may work against cost control, especially where compassion favors providing treatment that is not covered by a health plan.
Although these values seem relevant to providing medical care (and appear to be derived from principles used in medical ethics), more sophisticated concepts are necessary if they are to be incorporated into standards
that provide concrete guidance to MCOs.

Few business ethics texts even discuss organizations that deliver medical care. Most tend to focus on ethical principles for individual personal
conduct, rather than the actions or policies of an organization.[34] The
American College of Healthcare Executives (ACHE) has perhaps the best
code of ethics for the behavior of health care executives.[35] Its preamble
states that because "every management decision affects the health and
well-being of both individuals and communities," health care executives

"must safeguard and foster the rights, interests, and prerogatives of patients, clients or others served." Yet the code's normative responsibilities are primarily duties of honesty, such as conducting all professional activities with "honesty, integrity, respect, fairness, and good faith," being truthful and avoiding "information that is false, misleading, and deceptive or information that would create unreasonable expectation," avoiding "the exploitation of professional relationships for personal gain," and creating "institutional safeguards to prevent discriminatory organizational practices."

The ACHE code makes clear that executives have a responsibility to the organization as well as to patients, noting that they should respect the customs of patients "consistent with the organization's philosophy." Obligations to provide health care services may be limited by available resources. Although executives are to assure "a resource allocation process that considers ethical ramifications," the code does not indicate what ethical principles might be relevant.[36] The fundamental question for managers is whether their responsibilities to the organization supersede any responsibilities to the patients served by the organization. In other words, when the organization's financial needs conflict with the needs of patients, does the manager have an ethical obligation to give patient needs priority? Unfortunately, existing codes of ethics do not answer this question. Most imply that constraints on organizational resources also constrain obligations to patients.[37]

It is possible that ethical management principles would bar organizations from excluding physicians who generate high costs by providing appropriate care to their patients. After all, if the organization's mission is to provide appropriate care to its patient population, its employed or contracting physicians cannot be faulted for achieving that mission. This would support recommendations that MCOs evaluate physician performance solely on the basis of quality of care, without regard to the quantity or cost of services generated.[38] At the same time, the organization needs to preserve itself; and if the cost of providing appropriate care became unreasonable, even a principle requiring fair treatment of physicians might not override the financial imperative of self-preservation. In the absence of any standard for determining the proportion of resources that should be devoted to patient care and what an appropriate level of care should be, existing principles are not likely to resolve such conflicts. Moreover, fair treatment of physicians and employees would not require retaining subscribers whose illnesses were costly to treat. Thus, even ethical management principles are unlikely to prevent organizations from limiting medical benefits or excluding patients in the absence of other principles defining an obligation to provide care.

Even if codes of ethics for managers contained more specific normative principles, it is not clear how effective they would be in the face of countervailing financial pressure. No formal rules regulate the conduct of business managers. The ACHE's only sanction for violations of its code is expulsion from the ACHE, which does not necessarily affect an offender's ability to work. In contrast, a violation of the American Medical Association's *Principles of Medical Ethics*[39] could result in a complaint to the board of registration, which has the power to revoke a physician's license to practice medicine, even if such sanctions are rarely invoked in practice.

Ethical Obligations to Patients/Enrollees

Although patients may view their health plan as an assurance of medical care, their legal relationship to an MCO is based on contract principles developed for application in the marketplace of consumer goods. The conditions for an enforceable contract are an exchange of promises; a fair bargaining process (no coercion); and a meeting of the minds.[40] A relationship based on contract principles is fundamentally different from one based on trust or fiduciary obligations. For example, a physician has an ethical obligation to act in the patient's best interest, while a party to a contract need only perform according to the contract. Thus, in a contractual relationship, an MCO that does not provide care that is not promised in the contract does not treat patients unjustly, even if the care is necessary and appropriate.

While physicians have a duty to treat all patients equally, no contract principle requires that all contracts be the same. Thus, two patients with the same illness who are covered by different health plans may receive quite different treatment. In business ethics, the principle of honesty undoubtedly requires MCOs to inform prospective subscribers of the contract terms, but no principle insists that the contract contain specific benefits or be consistent with other contracts. Contract variations may violate some conceptions of justice, yet they are entirely consistent with market values and the goals of competition among health plans.

Fair competition is premised on the freedom of consumers to choose what goods and services to buy. In today's medical marketplace, consumer choice is advocated not only as a valuable freedom in itself, but also as a means to force MCOs to offer quality medical care. It is notable, therefore, that patient choice has all but disappeared from the goals of managed care.[41] If care is managed, then, by definition, the patient is not free to choose what care he or she gets. The *American Heritage Dictionary*, for example, defines *manage* as "to direct or control the use of; to exert control over; make submissive to one's authority, discipline, or persuasion."[42] The purpose of managing care is to eliminate choices that are wasteful, harmful, or too expensive. Patient choice is not always desirable from society's perspective, because patients sometimes make unwise choices and want unnecessary or even harmful treatment. Managed care's cost control mechanisms are designed to eliminate certain choices or to influence patients (by means of deductibles and copayments, for example) to choose specific (usually less expensive) types of care.[43] In the ideal world, good management will result in better care for patients, but it will not encourage patient choice.

Of course, managed care was never intended to promote patient choice of care. Rather, "choice" here is the choice of which health care plan to buy or "join."[44] If patients are consumers or customers, then the product is the health plan—that package of insured services paid for by the insurer, subject to deductibles, copayments, caps, and other limits. The organization's primary relationship to its patients is that of an insurer to an insured, not of a health care provider to a patient.[45] This is underscored by the insurance terminology for patients: subscribers, enrollees, or, most recently, covered lives.

Advocates of competition among health plans have argued that rational people will choose the health plan that suits their needs.[46] They assume that, when people choose a plan, they have deliberately and necessarily chosen its doctors, nurses, practice patterns, administrative procedures, and benefits package—everything about their health care. A choice to buy a cheaper plan entails assuming the risk that some services will not be covered. For this reason, they conclude, patients must live (or die) with their choices—that is, what the health plan contract provides. This conclusion is based on false assumptions. The most obvious is that people make rational choices about their health care. Even if people could make rational choices about their health care, there are at least three practical problems with assuming that choosing a health plan satisfies the requirements of choice.

First, most patients do not choose their health plans; their employers do. The vast majority of Americans with health insurance get it through their employers.[47] The insurer's primary customers are employers, not individual patients. A recent survey found that among companies with fewer than 50 employees and with employee health insurance, 86% offered only one plan.[48] Sixty percent of larger firms offered no choice. The number of employers who offer plans that are closed panel HMOs or limited panel preferred provider organizations (PPOs) is increasing.[49] MCO growth rates are expected to continue over the next few years as government programs like Medicare and Medicaid encourage more beneficiaries to join managed care plans.[50] Thus, the number of patients who have not merely a limited choice of plans, but no choice of plans, is increasing.

A recent Commonwealth Fund study of 3,000 employees in Boston, Los Angeles, and Miami found that 29% of respondents in managed care plans did not have the choice of enrolling in a FFS plan.[51] Those without such a choice reported more dissatisfaction with their plans than those who did.[52] Almost half of the employees had changed plans in the past three years, and, of those, nearly three-fourths did so involuntarily. Employees who changed health plans were often forced to change physicians as well: 48% of HMO enrollees and 29% of PPO enrollees, compared to 12% of FFS patients.

If patients are not choosing the plans they join, it cannot be said that they are freely entering into a contract by which they should be bound. Of course, they could "choose" not to join the employer's plan, but for many employees, such a "choice" is unaffordable. Furthermore, people whose employers do not offer health insurance may have little or no choice of plans they can afford.

A second reason why patients do not choose their health plans in practice is that patients rarely know exactly what benefits their plans offer when they must choose them. It is the rare patient who fully understands a benefit contract or appreciates what it means to "choose" a health plan. Contracts are frequently revised and may not even be available to subscribers in final form until several months into the contract year. Information about plans is ordinarily summarized in general terms in brochures distributed to employees or prospective subscribers.[53] Summaries are clearest on how to choose a physician, where services are and are not available, and the amounts of copayments and deductibles. Benefits are usually described generically as hospital care, physicians' services, and laboratory services, for example. Typically, mention is made of the fact that the plan covers "medically necessary" services, but subscribers may not appreciate that the term "medically necessary" serves as a limitation on coverage. It is often difficult to know what particular kinds of treatment are covered until a patient gets sick and needs specific services.[54] Then, it is too late: patients are not likely to be able to change plans at that time, either because they do not get sick during the annual plan enrollment period or because any new plan they join may exclude coverage for their now preexisting illness, at least for the period in which they need treatment. Thus, much of the information necessary for a rational choice is not available when the choice must be made.

Finally, many patients do not want to be bound by their contracts. Even if patients had perfect information and actually chose their health plans, they would not necessarily want contract exclusions enforced when they get sick. "A deal is a deal" is not a palatable response to a dying patient who cannot afford the recommended treatment. People who appear to be rational consumers when they enroll in a health plan may change their minds when they need treatment. Many are surprised to find that, contrary to their expectations, their health plan does not cover the care they need or desire.[55] Even those who might have appreciated that the plan would not cover certain kinds of care (or did not want to pay for it), such as experimental treatment, may consider the contract unfair if the experiment offers their only chance for survival.

Patients may be especially likely to consider benefit denials unfair in a competitive environment where a wide variety of health plans offer different benefits; patients know that other health plans provide the desired care to their subscribers. Even where benefits are the same, different insurers may interpret them differently, resulting in inconsistent benefit determinations.[56] Many patients are likely to perceive such variation not as healthy variety in a free marketplace, but as arbitrary and unfair rationing by their health plan.[57] Given recent publicity about high profits earned by many HMOs and about multimillion-dollar compensation paid to their chief executive officers, subscribers may also believe that different treatment is based on corporate greed, not on individual patient needs.[58] This is not to suggest that patients are entitled to whatever care they want, but rather that they may want it, regardless of what their health plan covers or of the likely effectiveness of the desired treatment.[59]

The circumstances in which individuals enroll in health plans today are significantly removed from the basic conditions for fair and enforceable contracts contemplated by law. Yet, in spite of deviations from the ideal, courts have not questioned the validity of such contracts. Neither have they hesitated to enforce contract exclusions (denying medical benefits to patients) when their terms were clear.[60] Although enforcement has been inconsistent, courts have most commonly refused to enforce coverage exclusions on the grounds that the contract language was ambiguous or the treatment at issue was not necessarily excluded by explicit language. Thus, it seems unlikely that patients could successfully claim that their health plans are invalid.

Of course, ethical standards may demand more than law requires. Thus, whether making patients abide by the terms of their health plans is fair or unfair depends on how fairly the plans themselves are structured. But what should count as a fair structure? What choices ought to be available to patients? Fundamentally, the search for standards of fairness is a quest for ethical principles that prescribe what kind of care patients should get. Medical ethics suggests that every patient is entitled to the best available care, but does not obligate anyone to provide that care if it is not paid for. Business ethics also does not obligate anyone to provide any particular care to anyone else, absent a contractual promise. An adequate answer requires more specific standards than either business or medical ethics offers.

Goals for Developing Standards

What might new ethical standards for MCOs look like? Several basic features appear necessary, but will require substantially more discussion, definition, and clarification than can be offered here.

First, ethical standards for MCOs should recognize the organizations' medical responsibilities as well as their business functions. The organization has responsibility—as an organization—for providing health care to individual enrollees, and this responsibility should not be delegable to individuals, even though officers and staff should remain bound by their personal ethical obligations. MCOs should be held directly accountable to enrollees for the scope and quality of patient care, because patients are not customers in the usual sense. Because the MCO's mission is to finance and provide quality medical care, its business structures, policies, and practices should facilitate and not hinder good care. Indeed, ethical standards should give priority to MCO's medical mission.

Second, organizational standards should reflect ethical principles that apply to all human endeavors, such as fairness, honesty, and truthfulness, respect for persons, and justice. The principle of justice, which governs resource allocation, is especially relevant to MCOs because the very nature of managed care requires allocating resources for the benefit of all members of a group. MCOs must marshal sufficient resources (both human and financial) to care for an entire patient population. In this respect, MCOs differ from other commercial enterprises that do not attempt to allocate their products or services among their potential customers. While physicians may act as patient advocates, the organization's purpose is to ensure that *all* of its enrollees receive appropriate care. Obvious potential conflicts arise between being fair to a population and being fair to an individual patient. But reaching acceptable solutions is more likely when decisions are based on ethical principles of justice and respect for persons than when they are perceived to be based on financial self-interest.

Of course, reasonable people disagree on what justice requires and on what counts as a just allocation of resources.[61] A standard that allocates benefits according to patient need is as plausible as one that eliminates expensive, experimental therapies in order to provide more preventive services. Some proponents of market competition in health care also adopt a libertarian view of justice that does not require any particular distribution of services. In this view, the principles of fair contracting are sufficient to create a just allocation of resources, without regard to who receives what services or why. This latter approach, in effect, argues against any ethical standard that seeks to achieve a more equal distribution of services or benefits.

An even greater difficulty with just allocation as an ethical standard for MCOs is that it applies only to the organization itself. Although one MCO may produce a just distribution of resources across its own subscribers, it does not affect those in other plans or those without health insurance, so that the allocating of resources throughout society may remain quite unjust. One organization cannot be expected to solve the inequities of society as a whole, but society should recognize that organizations whose standards are entirely inward-looking are not likely to produce a fairer health care system.

The principles of honesty and fairness suggest that MCOs should fully and completely disclose the terms and conditions of the contracts they offer, especially in a market system that depends on consumer demand. At a minimum, this requires telling current and potential enrollees (and the public) what the plan does and does not provide and the specific conditions in which services will be made available, and ensuring that patients are not coerced into a particular plan.[62] An obligation on the MCO's part for even more extensive disclosure is supported by traditional business ethics and assumptions about market transactions. Fair competition requires informed consumers. Disclosure is a competitive market method of promoting informed consumer choice.

Full disclosure is also supported, analogously, by the doctrine of informed consent.[63] If a subscriber is validly to consent to join a health plan (and to be bound by its terms), then the MCO—the entity with the relevant information—should have a duty to disclose all information relevant to the subscriber's decision. This should include detailed information on the specific treatments that are and are not covered for particular medical conditions, the criteria for making decisions about new or innovative therapies, the MCO's history of approving or denying claims for treatment, and procedures for challenging treatment denials. In addition, the MCO should disclose all financial arrangements with providers, including affiliated physicians and hospitals, and the organization's officers and employees.[64] Standard formats for presenting information should be developed to enable consumers to compare different health plans. The MCO should also ensure that its officers, employees, and health care practitioners are equally open and honest with patients. Full disclosure is intended to move the relationship between MCOs and patients closer to one of fair bargaining, so that patients can actually begin to choose.[65]

There are limits to the utility of information disclosure, however.[66] Not everyone will see or understand the information provided. More important, many consumers do not have the freedom to act on the information or to bargain at all. Their employer may offer only one plan and they may not be able to afford the plan they prefer. The current market does not include any mechanism for such consumers to pressure MCOs to change their policies.[67] Thus, full disclosure is necessary, but insufficient to foster a fair contractual relationship.

MCOs that distinguish themselves by adhering to ethical standards may find that they are penalized in the marketplace. For most commercial enterprises, customer satisfaction produces increased revenues and profits and higher stock values. Patient satisfaction, however, may be associated with more services that cost a for-profit MCO revenues and reduce stock prices. A competitive market is likely to discourage MCOs from seeking subscribers who are likely to need expensive medical care (or from contracting with their physicians). This means that a competitive market will not provide universal health insurance coverage. Some regulation may be necessary to permit MCOs to compete without abandoning their ethical standards. For example, were all companies required to enroll individuals regardless of their medical conditions (assuming a fair distribution of either high risk patients or premium adjustments, with or without financial assistance from government), MCOS would be free to compete on quality of care, including patient satisfaction. Universal coverage would undoubtedly reduce the feasible profit margin for all companies, but the pressure to sacrifice patient welfare for cost control would be substantially diminished. In such circumstances, ethical standards promoting patient welfare could enhance a company's competitive position. Thus, a regulated market that removes or reduces incentives to compete for profits is more likely to encourage the adoption of ethical standards that protect patients.

Conclusion

MCOS combine insurance, management, and health care delivery. They face conflicts, between their financial incentives and their mission (or potential ethical duty) to provide appropriate care, that are analogous to the conflicts faced by physicians in MCOS. The difference between the organizations and the physicians (and other professionals) is that neither the manager nor the organization has any significant history of ethical obligations that counter inappropriate financial incentives. Patients and physicians may wish to judge MCOS by ethical standards that were created for individual physicians and nurses, but the market in which MCOS operate does not use those standards. Those who argue that MCOS should operate like efficient businesses in the competitive marketplace are, in effect, arguing for no standards at all. A free market approach stresses organizing and delivering health care in an economically efficient, value-free way. This effectively precludes the imposition of normative values on MCOS.

In absence of standards that address MCOS' business and medical functions, we may be left with two incompatible sets of standards—one for business and one for medicine. Scholars have begun to rethink conceptions of medical ethics for physicians in MCOS. It is time to rethink business ethics for MCOS. If business ethics do not recognize an organizational commitment to patient welfare, conflicts between physicians and managers, and managers and patients, may be exacerbated, putting financial power against patient welfare. In such circumstances, it is not cynical to fear that financial pressure may overwhelm patient welfare, leaving companies who risk too much money to provide services to patients at a competitive disadvantage or out of business.

MCOs should not have to choose between ethics and money, but they do need a different set of standards from those of ordinary commercial enterprises. The challenge is to formulate new standards that apply to organizations, not just individuals, and that recognize and reconcile their business and medical functions. If such standards are to be more than idealistic goals, however, it may be necessary to regulate the market to make it possible for organizations to put such standards into practice.

Notes

1   Erik Eckholm, "While Congress Remains Silent, Health Care Transforms Itself," *New York Times*, Dec. 18, 1994, at 34.

2   John K. Iglehart, "The American Health Care System—Managed Care," *N. Engl. J. Med.*, 327 (1992): 743–47.

3   Marc A. Rodwin, "Conflicts in Managed Care," *N. Engl. J. Med.*, 332 (1995): 604–07.

4   Marc A. Rodwin, *Medicine, Money & Morals: Physicians' Conflicts of Interest* (New York: Oxford University Press, 1993); and Peter Franks, Carolyn M. Clancy, and Paul A. Nutting, "Gatekeeping Revisited—Protecting Patients from Overtreatment," *N. Engl. J. Med.*, 327 (1992): 424–29.

5   Edmund D. Pellegrino, "Words *Can* Hurt You: Some Reflections on the Metaphors of Managed Care," *Journal of the American Board of Family Practice*, 7 (1994): 505–10.

6   Committee on Child Health Financing, American Academy of Pediatrics, "Guiding Principles for Managed Care Arrangements for the Health Care of Infants, Children, Adolescents, and Young Adults," *Pediatrics*, 95 (1995): 613–15; Council on Ethical and Judicial Affairs, American Medical Association, "Ethical Issues in Managed Care," *JAMA*, 271 (1994): 1668–70; Mark H. Waymack, "Health Care as a Business: The Ethic of Hippocrates versus the Ethic of Managed Care," *Business & Professional Ethics Journal*, 9, nos. 3–4 (1990: 69–78; and Susan M. Wolf, "Health Care Reform and the Future of Physician Ethics," *Hastings Center Report*, 24, no. 2 (1994): 28–41.

7   Carolyn M. Clancy and Howard Brody, "Managed Care—Jekyll or Hyde?," *JAMA*, 273 (1995): 338–39.

8   The percentage of MCOs that are for-profit companies grew from 18% in 1982 to 67% in 1988. See Karen Davis et al., *Health Care Cost Containment* (Baltimore: Johns Hopkins University Press, 1990).

9   The White House Domestic Policy Council, *The President's Health Security Plan: The Clinton Blueprint* (New York: Times Books, 1993): at 11–12.

10 As Sager has noted, managed care, in the form of employee group health organizations, was considered a radical (even socialist) innovation before and after World War II. See Alan Sager, "Reforming Managed Care: More Benefits—Fewer Costs," presented at the conference "Ethics of Managed Care: Values, Conflicts, and Resolutions," Boston University

School of Public Health, Boston, Massachusetts, December 9, 1994. Group Health of Puget Sound, the Health Insurance Plan of New York, and the Kaiser-Permanente Medical Care Program have provided comprehensive care at a relatively reasonable cost to large groups of employees for at least fifty years. See John G. Smillie, *Can Physicians Manage the Quality and Costs of Medical Care? The Story of the Permanente Group* (New York: McGraw-Hill, 1991).

11 Theodore R. Marmor and Jonathan Oberlander, "A Citizen's Guide to the Healthcare Reform Debate," *Yale Journal on Regulation*, 11 (1994): 495–506.

12 Stephen M. Shortell, Robin R. Gillies, and David A. Anderson, "The New World of Managed Care: Creating Organized Delivery Systems, *Health Affairs*, 13, no. 4 (1994): 46–64; and Alain C. Enthoven, "The History and Principles of Managed Competition," *Health Affairs*, 12, supp. (1993): 24–48.

13 Paul Starr, "Looks Who's Talking Health Care Reform Now," *New York Times Magazine*, Sept. 3, 1995, at 42–43.

14 R. H. Miller and Harold S. Luft, "Managed Care Plan Performance since 1980: A Literature Analysis," *JAMA*, 271 (1995): 1512–19.

15 Congressional Budget Office, *The Effects of Managed Care and Managed Competition, CBO Memorandum* (Washington, D.C.: Congressional Budget Office, Feb. 1995); Theodore R. Marmor and Jerry L. Mashaw, "Conceptualizing, Estimating, and Reforming Fraud, Waste, and Abuse in Healthcare Spending," *Yale Journal on Regulation*, 11 (1994): 455–94; William B. Schwartz and Daniel N. Mendelson, "Eliminating Waste and Inefficiency Can Do Little to Contain Costs," *Health Affairs*, 13, no. 1 (1994): 223–35; and Henry Aaron and William B. Schwartz, "Rationing Health Care: The Choice before Us," *Science*, 247 (1990): 418–202.

16 See Iglehart, *supra* note 2.

17 Institute of Medicine, Bradford H. Gray and Marilyn J. Fields, eds., *Controlling Costs and Changing Patient Care? The Role of Utilization Management* (Washington, D.C.: National Academy Press, 1989); Alan L. Hillman, Mark V. Pauly, and Joseph J. Kerstein, "How Do Financial Incentives Affect Physicians' Clinical Decisions and the Financial Performance of Health Maintenance Organizations?," *N. Engl. J. Med.*, 321 (1989): 87–92; and Rodwin, *supra* note 4.

18 Donald W. Light, "The Practice and Ethics of Risk-Rated Health Insurance," *JAMA*, 267 (1992): 2503–08.

19 Several states have considered legislation prohibiting insurers from excluding coverage of preexisting medical conditions (completely or for a limited time period). In general, the insurance industry has opposed such legislation.

20 James Morone, "The Ironic Flaw in Health Care Competition: The Politics of Markets," in Richard J. Arnould et al., eds., *Competitive Approaches to Health Care Reform* (Washington, D.C.: Urban Institute Press, 1993): 207–22; Gerald W. Grumet, "Health Care Rationing through Inconvenience: The Third Party's Secret Weapon," *N. Engl. J. Med.*, 321 (1989): 607–11; U.S. Inspector General, *Beneficiary Perspectives of Medicare Risk HMOS* (Washington, D.C.: Dept. of Health and Human Services, OEI-06-91-00730, 1995); and Robert Blendon, *Sick People in Managed Care Have Difficulty Getting Services and Treatment* (Princeton: Robert Wood Johnson Foundation, 1995).

21 Wendy K. Mariner, "Patients' Rights after Health Care Reform: Who Decides What Is Medically Necessary?," *American Journal of Public Health*, 84 (1994): 1515–20.

22   U.S. Congress, Office of Technology Assessment, *Identifying Health Technologies That Work: Searching for Evidence* (Washington, D.C.: Government Printing Office, OTA-H-608, Sept. 1994); and Wendy K. Mariner, "Outcomes Assessment in Health Care Reform: Promise and Limitations," *American Journal of Law & Medicine*, 20 (1994): 37–57.

23   Tom Beauchamp and LeRoy Walters, *Contemporary Issues in Bioethics* (Belmont: Wadsworth, 4th ed., 1994). The concept of medical ethics itself is subject to different interpretations. See Michael A. Grodin, "Introduction: The Historical and Philosophical Roots of Bioethics," in Michael A. Grodin, ed., *Meta Medical Ethics: The Philosophical Foundations of Bioethics* (Dordrecht: Kluwer, 1995): at 1–26.

24   See Wolf, *supra* note 6.

25   George J. Annas, "Transferring the Ethical Hot Potato," *Hastings Center Report*, 17, no. 1 (1987): 20–21. With respect to whether corporations in general are moral entities, compare Milton Friedman, "The Social Responsibility of Business Is to Increase its Profits," *New York Times Magazine*, Sept. 13, 1970, at 32–33, 122, 124, 126; Herbert A. Simon, *Administrative Behavior* (New York: Free Press, 1965) (arguing that corporations cannot be held morally responsible); and John Ladd, "Morality and the Ideal of Rationality in Formal Organizations," *The Monist*, 54 (1970): 488–516 (arguing for corporate responsibility). For general discussions of the debate, see Peter A. French, *Collective and Corporate Responsibility* (New York: Columbia University Press, 1984); and Hugh Curtler, ed., *Shame, Responsibility and the Corporation* (New York: Haven, 1986).

26   Richard T. DeGeorge, *Business Ethics* (New York: Macmillan, 4th ed., 1995): at 127.

27   Legal obligations have been a significant source of ethical standards for business. See Paul Steidlmeier, *People and Profits: The Ethics of Capitalism* (Englewood Cliffs: Prentice Hall, 1992): at 14; and John R. Boatright, *Ethics and the Conduct of Business* (Englewood Cliffs: Prentice Hall, 1993): at 386. Federal antitrust legislation, such as the Sherman Act and the Robinson-Patman Act, were arguably efforts to impose ethical standards of fair competition on industry, and law is often seen as the "guardian of business ethics." See Verne E. Henderson, *What's Ethical in Business* (New York: McGraw-Hill, 1992): at 7.

28   Daniel P. Sulmasy, "Physicians, Cost Control and Ethics," *Annals of Internal Medicine*, 116 (1992): 920–26; Gail Povar and John Moreno, "Hippocrates and the Health Maintenance Organization," *Annals of Internal Medicine*, 109 (1988): 419–24; Council on Ethical and Judicial Affairs, *supra* note 6; Pellegrino, *supra* note 5; and Wolf, *supra* note 6.

29   Lester C. Thurow, "Medicine Versus Economics," *N. Engl. J. Med.*, 313 (1985): 611–14.

30   See, for example, DeGeorge, *supra* note 26; James P. Wilbur, *The Moral Foundations of Business Practice* (Lanham: University Press of America, 1992); Ronald M. Green, *The Ethical Manager: A New Method for Business Ethics* (New York: Macmillan, 1994); Ronald Berenbeim, *Corporate Ethics* (New York: Conference Board, 1992); Karen Paul, ed., *Business Environment and Business Ethics* (Cambridge: Ballinger, 1987); and Henderson, *supra* note 27.

31   See Boatright, *supra* note 27, at 386; and DeGeorge, *supra* note 26.

32   Stanley Joel Reiser, "The Ethical Life of Health Care Organizations," *Hastings Center Report*, 24, no. 6 (1994): 28–35.

33   See DeGeorge, *supra* note 26. Steidlmeier has summarized American business values as follows: "(1) protecting the interests of property owners by promoting efficiency, reducing costs, and thereby increasing profits; (2) encouraging respect for the rights of property owners; (3) refraining from anticompetitive activities; (4) guarding the freedom of labor,

owners, and customers; (5) discouraging government interference; (6) developing personal honesty, responsibility and industriousness; and (7) encouraging private contributions to charity." See Steidlmeier, *supra* note 27.

34 See, for example, Kurt Darr, *Ethics in Health Services Management* (Baltimore: Health Professions Press, 2d ed., 1993), which is directed at developing a personal ethic for individual managers.

35 American College of Healthcare Executives, *Code of Ethics* (1988).

36 The American College of Health Care Administrators' *Code of Ethics* requires the administrator to "strive to provide to all those entrusted to his or her care the highest quality of appropriate services possible *in light of resources or other constraints.*" See the American College of Health Care Administrators, *Code of Ethics* (1989) (emphasis added). Even the Joint Commission on Accreditation of Healthcare Organizations, which requires hospitals to have a mechanism for considering ethical issue in patient care, qualifies its requirement by providing that the hospital reasonably respond to a patient's need for treatment "within the hospital's capacity." See Joint Commission on Accreditation of Healthcare Organizations, *1995 Accreditation Manual for Hospitals*, Vol. 1, *Standards* (Oakbrook Terrace: JCAHO, 1994).

37 The Group Health Association of America has proposed some standards for managed care and health plans, but these deal with financial solvency requirements (common in insurance regulation), patient confidentiality, and some consumer protections. See John K. Iglehart, "The Struggle between Managed Care and Fee-for-Service Practice," *N. Engl. J. Med.*, 331 (1994): 63–67.

38 See Council on Ethical and Judicial Affairs, *supra* note 6.

39 American Medical Association, *Principles of Medical Ethics* (Chicago: American Medical Association, 1980).

40 Joseph M. Perillo, *Corbin on Contracts* (St. Paul: West, vol. 1, 1993).

41 MCOs are increasingly offering preferred provider or point of service plans that permit enrollees to obtain service outside the plan's network of providers for a larger copayment or deductible. Such plans appear to be a response to enrollee demand for greater freedom to choose physicians and services.

42 *American Heritage Dictionary* (Boston: Houghton Mifflin, 1978): at 792.

43 Health plans that offer services through independent practice association (IPAS) preserve greater choice of physicians for enrollees than do staff model HMOs, for example. Historically, however, IPAS have produced smaller cost savings for health plans. See Miller and Luft, *supra* note 14.

44 Alain C. Enthoven and Richard Kronick, "A Consumer-Choice Health Plan for the 1990's: Universal Health Insurance in a System Designed to Promote Quality and Economy," *N. Engl. J. Med.*, 320 (1989): 29–37.

45 Of course, most MCOs also provide health care through providers in a widening array of organizational structures, including staff model HMOs, group practice HMOs, networks of IPAS, or other integrated services and preferred provider organizations.

46 Paul Starr, "The Framework of Health Care Reform," *N. Engl. J. Med.*, 329 (1993): 1666–72; Enthoven and Kronick, *supra* note 44; Mark A. Hall and Gerard F. Anderson, "Health Insurers' Assessment of Medical Necessity," *University of Pennsylvania Law Review*, 140 (1992): 1637–712; Paul T. Menzel, *Strong Medicine: The Ethical Rationing of Health Care* (New York: Oxford University Press, 1990); and David Eddy, "Clinical Decision Making:

From Theory to Practice—Connecting Value and Costs—Whom Do We Ask and What Do We Ask Them?," *JAMA*, 264 (1990): 1737–39.

47 Employee Benefit Research Institute, *Sources of Health Insurance and Characteristics of the Uninsured: Analysis of the March 1993 Current Population Survey* (Washington, D.C.: EBRI, Jan. 1994).

48 Joel C. Cantor, Stephen H. Long, and M. Susan Marquis, "Private Employer-Based Health Insurance in Ten States," *Health Affairs*, 14, no. 2 (1995): 199–211. Smaller employers were more likely than larger to offer a FFS plan, but such plans were more likely to cover fewer benefits and to exclude preexisting conditions. Only about half of the smaller employers offered any health insurance at all.

49 Deborah Chollet, "Employer-Based Health Insurance in a Changing Work Force," *Health Affairs*, 13, no. 1 (1994): 327–36.

50 Christopher Georges, "Medicare Drive toward Managed-Care System Could Turn Out to Produce a Costly Success," *Wall Street Journal*, July 31, 1995, at 16; and John K. Iglehart, "Medicaid and Managed Care," *N. Engl. J. Med.*, 322 (1995): 1727–31. Some states, like Tennessee, Florida, and New York, have reported problems in moving Medicaid beneficiaries quickly into some managed care plans. See Ian Fisher, "Forced Marriage of Medicaid and Managed Care Hits Snags," *New York Times*, Aug. 28, 1995, at B1, B5; and Martin Gottlieb, "The Managed Care Cure-All Shows Its Flaws and Potential," *New York Times*, Oct. 1, 1995, at 1, 16.

51 Karen Davis et al., "Choice Matters: Enrollees' Views of Their Health Plans," *Health Affairs*, 14, no. 2 (1995): 99–112.

52 The Commonwealth Fund Survey found that among respondents who reported a serious illness, 45% of those in FFS medicine rated their plans as excellent, compared to 33% of those in managed care. *Id.*

53 The Employee Retirement Income Security Act, 29 U.S.C.S. §§1021–25 (1995), which governs employee group health insurance plans offered by employers, requires only that employees receive a summary of the plan, not the contract itself.

54 Describing covered benefits in detail would require extensive lists because appropriate treatment often depends significantly on individual medical conditions. See Ira Mark Ellman and Mark A. Hall, "Redefining the Terms of Insurance to Accommodate Varying Consumer Risk Preferences," *American Journal of Law & Medicine*, 20 (1994): 187–201.

55 Recent examples of patients who claimed their health plan should have covered various treatments are described in a series of articles by Michael A. Hiltzik, David R. Olmos, and Barbara Marsh in the *Los Angeles Times*, Aug. 27–31, 1995.

56 U.S. General Accounting Office, *Medicare Part B: Inconsistent Denial Rates for Medical Necessity across Six Carriers* (Washington, D.C.: GAO, GAO/T-PEMD-94-17, 1994); and General Accounting Office, *Medicare Part B: Regional Variation in Denial Rates for Medical Necessity* (Washington, D.C.: GAO, GAO/PEMD-95-10, 1994).

57 Wendy K. Mariner, "Rationing Health Care and the Need for Credible Scarcity: Why Americans Can't Say No," *American Journal of Public Health*, 85 (1995): 1439–45.

58 George Anders, "HMOs Pile Up Billions in Cash, Try to Decide What to Do with It," *Wall Street Journal*, Dec. 21, 1994, at A1, A5; and Milt Freudenheim, "Penny-pinching H.M.O.'s Showed Their Generosity in Executive Paychecks," *New York Times*, Apr. 11, 1995, at D1, D4. In remarks to Congress on August 30, 1995, H. Ross Perot was reported to say, "If someone were to ask me what is my principal concern about H.M.O.'s, it's the giant

concentration of power; it's the giant salaries. . . . You know, that doesn't look good to me." See Robert Pear, "Perot Tells Senate Committee It's Time to Get Experts' Opinion on Reining in Medicare," *New York Times*, Aug. 31, 1995, at B13.

59 See Mariner, *supra* note 57.

60 See, for example, *Fuja v. Benefit Trust Life Ins. Co.*, 18 F.3d 1405 (7th Cir. 1994).

61 For summaries of different conceptions of justice with respect to allocating health care resources, see John F. Kilner, "Allocation of Health-Care Resources," in Warren Thomas Reich, ed., *Encyclopedia of Bioethics* (New York: Simon & Schuster, vol. 4, 1995): at 1067–84; and President's Commission for the Study of Ethical Problems in Medicine and Biomedical and Behavioral Research, *Securing Access to Health Care: Report on the Ethical Implications of Differences in the Availability of Health Services* (Washington, D.C.: President's Commission, 1983).

62 Anderson et al. have recommended objective assessments of technologies and therapies and better education to ensure that patients know what they are buying. Gerald F. Anderson, Mark A. Hall, and Earl P. Steinberg, "Medical Technology Assessment and Practice Guidelines: Their Day in Court," *American Journal of Public Health*, 83 (1993): 1635–39.

63 Ruth R. Faden and Tom L. Beauchamp, *A History and Theory of Informed Consent* (New York: Oxford University Press, 1986).

64 Ironically, capitation of physicians—the financial arrangement that has prompted the most concern about ethical standards—may be the least problematic method of payment. This is because capitation permits the MCO to avoid micromanaging patient care decisions in order to control costs. When the risk of financial loss is shifted to the physician, an MCO's financial self-interest rarely conflicts with patient welfare. It is the physician who faces a potential conflict. Physicians have a longer history of personal obligations to patients defined by medical ethics. Nonetheless, because the MCO is responsible for patient care, it should have a responsibility to calculate capitation payments that adequately provide for its patients. In addition, the MCO may be obligated to create different physician payment arrangements that reduce the potential conflict of interest.

65 Several states have introduced legislation to require the disclosure of certain information by MCOs, but the industry has generally opposed such regulation. Michael A. Hiltzik and David R. Olmos, "State Widely Criticized for Regulation of HMOs," *Los Angeles Times*, Aug. 28, 1995, at A1.

66 See Rodwin, *supra* note 4, at 212–22.

67 Yarmolinsky has noted, "Patients may be the only consumers who have to seek permission from someone else in order to obtain services." See Adam Yarmolinsky, "Supporting the Patient," *N. Engl. J. Med.*, 332 (1995): 602–03. In some instances, employees may be able to persuade their employers to offer a different health plan or to have the employer negotiate with an MCO to change the terms of the plan.

The Prostitute, the Playboy, and the Poet: Rationing Schemes for Organ Transplantation

George J. Annas

In the public debate about the availability of heart and liver transplants, the issue of rationing on a massive scale has been credibly raised for the first time in United States medical care. In an era of scarce resources, the eventual arrival of such a discussion was, of course, inevitable.[1] Unless we decide to ban heart and liver transplantation, or make them available to everyone, some rationing scheme must be used to choose among potential transplant candidates. The debate has existed throughout the history of medical ethics. Traditionally it has been stated as a choice between saving one of two patients, both of whom require the immediate assistance of the only available physician to survive.

National attention was focused on decisions regarding the rationing of kidney dialysis machines when they were first used on a limited basis in the late 1960s. As one commentator described the debate within the medical profession: "Shall machines or organs go to the sickest, or to the ones with most promise of recovery; on a first-come, first-served basis; to the most 'valuable' patient (based on wealth, education, position, what?); to the one with the most dependents; to women and children first; to those who can pay; to whom? Or should lots be cast, impersonally and uncritically?"[2]

In Seattle, Washington, an anonymous screening committee was set up to pick who among competing candidates would receive the life-saving technology. One lay member of the screening committee is quoted as saying:

> The choices were hard . . . I remember voting against a young woman who was a known prostitute. I found I couldn't vote for her, rather

George J. Annas, "The Prostitute, the Playboy and the Poet: Rationing Schemes for Organ Transplantation," from *American Journal of Public Health*, vol. 75, 187–189. © 1985. Reprinted by permission of American Public Health Association and George J. Annas.

than another candidate, a young wife and mother. I also voted against a young man who, until he learned he had renal failure, had been a ne'er do-well, a real playboy. He promised he would reform his character, go back to school, and so on, if only he were selected for treatment. But I felt I'd lived long enough to know that a person like that won't really do what he was promising at the time.[3]

When the biases and selection criteria of the committee were made public, there was a general negative reaction against this type of arbitrary device. Two experts reacted to the "numbing accounts of how close to the surface lie the prejudices and mindless cliches that pollute the committee's deliberations," by concluding that the committee was "measuring persons in accordance with its own middle-class values." The committee process, they noted, ruled out "creative nonconformists" and made the Pacific Northwest "no place for a Henry David Thoreau with bad kidneys."[4]

To avoid having to make such explicit, arbitrary, "social worth" determinations, the Congress, in 1972, enacted legislation that provided federal funds for virtually all kidney dialysis and kidney transplantation procedures in the United States.[5] This decision, however, simply served to postpone the time when identical decisions will have to be made about candidates for heart and liver transplantation in a society that does not provide sufficient financial and medical resources to provide all "suitable" candidates with the operation.

There are four major approaches to rationing scarce medical resources: the market approach; the selection committee approach; the lottery approach; and the "customary" approach.[1]

The Market Approach

The market approach would provide an organ to everyone who could pay for it with their own funds or private insurance. It puts a very high value on individual rights, and a very low value on equality and fairness. It has properly been criticized on a number of bases, including that the transplant technologies have been developed and are supported with public funds, that medical resources used for transplantation will not be available for higher priority care, and that financial success alone is an insufficient justification for demanding a medical procedure. Most telling is its complete lack of concern for fairness and equity.[6]

A "bake sale" or charity approach that requires the less financially fortunate to make public appeals for funding is demeaning to the individuals involved, and to society as a whole. Rationing by financial ability says we do not believe in equality, but believe that a price can and should be placed on human life and that it should be paid by the individual whose life is at stake. Neither belief is tolerable in a society in which income is inequitably distributed.

The Committee Selection Process

The Seattle Selection Committee is a model of the committee process. Ethics Committees set up in some hospitals to decide whether or not certain handicapped newborn infants should be given medical care may represent another.[7] These committees have developed because it was seen as unworkable or unwise to explicitly set forth the criteria on which selection decisions would be made. But only two results are possible, as Professor Guido Calabresi has pointed out: either a pattern of decision making will develop or it will not. If a pattern does develop (e.g., in Seattle, the imposition of middle-class values), then it can be articulated and those decision "rules" codified and used directly, without resort to the committee. If a pattern does not develop, the committee is vulnerable to the charge that it is acting arbitrarily, or dishonestly, and therefore cannot be permitted to continue to make such important decisions.[1]

In the end, public designation of a committee to make selection decisions on vague criteria will fail because it too closely involves the state and all members of society in explicitly preferring specific individuals over others, and in devaluing the interests those others have in living. It thus directly undermines, as surely as the market system does, society's view of equality and the value of human life.

The Lottery Approach

The lottery approach is the ultimate equalizer which puts equality ahead of every other value. This makes it extremely attractive, since all comers have an equal chance at selection regardless of race, color, creed, or financial status. On the other hand, it offends our notions of efficiency and fairness since it makes *no* distinctions among such things as the strength of the desires of the candidates, their potential survival, and their quality of life. In this sense it is a mindless method of trying to solve society's dilemma which is caused by its unwillingness or inability to spend enough resources to make a lottery unnecessary. By making this macro spending decision evident to all, it also undermines society's view of the priceless-ness of human life. A first-come, first-served system is a type of natural lottery since referral to a transplant program is generally random in time. Nonetheless, higher income groups have quicker access to referral networks and thus have an inherent advantage over the poor in a strict first-come, first-served system.[8,9]

The Customary Approach

Society has traditionally attempted to avoid explicitly recognizing that we are making a choice not to save individual lives because it is too expensive to do so. As long as such decisions are not explicitly acknowledged, they can be tolerated by society. For example, until recently there was said to be a general understanding among general practitioners in Britain that individuals over age 55 suffering from end-stage kidney disease not be referred for dialysis or transplant. In 1984, however, this unwritten practice became highly publicized, with figures that showed a rate of new cases of end-stage kidney disease treated in Britain at 40 per million (versus the U.S. figure of 80 per million) resulting in 1,500–3,000 "unnecessary deaths" annually.[10] This has, predictably, led to movements to enlarge the National Health Service budget to expand dialysis services to meet this need, a more socially acceptable solution than permitting the now publicly recognized situation to continue.

In the United States, the customary approach permits individual physicians to select their patients on the basis of medical criteria or clinical suitability. This, however, contains much hidden social worth criteria. For example, one criterion, common in the transplant literature, requires an individual to have sufficient family support for successful aftercare. This discriminates against individuals without families and those who have become alienated from their families. The criterion may be relevant, but it is hardly medical.

Similar observations can be made about medical criteria that include IQ, mental illness, criminal records, employment, indigency, alcoholism, drug addiction, or geographical location. Age is perhaps more difficult, since it may be impressionistically related to outcome. But it is not medically logical to assume that an individual who is 49 years old is necessarily a better medical candidate for a transplant than one who is 50 years old. Unless specific examination of the characteristics of older persons that make them less desirable candidates is undertaken, such a cut off is arbitrary, and thus devalues the lives of older citizens. The same can be said of blanket exclusions of alcoholics and drug addicts.

In short, the customary approach has one great advantage for society and one great disadvantage: it gives us the illusion that we do not have to make choices; but the cost is mass deception, and when this deception is uncovered, we must deal with it either by universal entitlement or by choosing another method of patient selection.

A Combination of Approaches

A socially acceptable approach must be fair, efficient, and reflective of important social values. The most important values at stake in organ transplantation are fairness itself, equity in the sense of equality, and the value of life. To promote efficiency, it is important that no one receive a transplant unless they want one and are likely to obtain significant benefit from it in the sense of years of life at a reasonable level of functioning.

Accordingly, it is appropriate for there to be an initial screening process that is based *exclusively* on medical criteria designed to measure the probability of a successful transplant, that is, one in which the patient survives for at least a number of years and is rehabilitated. There is room in medical criteria for social worth judgments, but there is probably no way to avoid this completely. For example, it has been noted that "in many respects social and medical criteria are inextricably intertwined" and that therefore medical criteria might "exclude the poor and disadvantaged because health and socioeconomic status are highly interdependent."[11] Roger Evans gives an example. In the End Stage Renal Disease Program, "those of lower socioeconomic status are likely to have multiple comorbid health conditions such as diabetes, hepatitis, and hypertension" making them both less desirable candidates and more expensive to treat.[11]

To prevent the gulf between the haves and have nots from widening, we must make every reasonable attempt to develop medical criteria that are objective and independent of social worth categories. One minimal way to approach this is to require that medical screening be reviewed and approved by an ethics committee with significant public representation, filed with a public agency, and made readily available to the public for comment. In the event that more than one hospital in a state or region is offering a particular transplant service, it would be most fair and efficient for the individual hospitals to perform the initial medical screening themselves (based on the uniform, objective criteria), but to have all subsequent nonmedical selection done by a method approved by a single selection committee composed of representatives of all hospitals engaged in a particular transplant procedure, as well as significant representation of the public at large.

As this implies, after the medical screening is performed, there may be more acceptable candidates in the "pool" than there are organs or surgical teams to go around. Selection among waiting candidates will then be necessary. This situation occurs now in kidney transplantation, but since the organ matching is much more sophisticated than in hearts and livers (permitting much more precise matching of organ and recipient), and since dialysis permits individuals to wait almost indefinitely for an organ without risking death, the situations are not close enough to permit use of the same matching criteria. On the other hand, to the extent that organs are specifically tissue- and size-matched and fairly distributed to the best matched candidate, the organ distribution system itself will resemble a natural lottery.

When a pool of acceptable candidates is developed, a decision about who gets the next available, suitable organ must be made. We must choose between using a conscious, value-laden, social worth selection criterion (including a committee to make the actual choice), or some type of random device. In view of the unacceptability and arbitrariness of social worth criteria being applied, implicitly or explicitly, by committee, this method is neither viable nor proper. On the other hand, strict adherence to a lottery might create a situation where an individual who has only a one-in-four chance of living five years with a transplant (but who could survive another six months without one) would get an organ before an individual who could survive as long or longer, but who will die within days or hours if he or she is not immediately transplanted. Accordingly, the most reasonable approach seems to be to allocate organs on a first-come, first-served basis to members of the pool but permit individuals to "jump" the queue if the second level selection committee believes they are in immediate danger of death (but still have a reasonable prospect for long-term survival with a transplant) and the person who would otherwise get the organ can survive long enough to be reasonably assured that he or she will be able to get another organ.

The first-come, first-served method of basic selection (after a medical screen) seems the preferred method because it most closely approximates the randomness of a straight lottery without the obviousness of making equity the only promoted value. Some unfairness is introduced by the fact that the more wealthy and medically astute will likely get into the pool first, and thus be ahead in line, but this advantage should decrease sharply as public awareness of the system grows. The possibility of unfairness is also inherent in permitting individuals to jump the queue, but some flexibility needs to be retained in the system to permit it to respond to reasonable contingencies.

We will have to face the fact that should the resources devoted to organ transplantation be limited (as they are now and are likely to be in the future), at some point it is likely that significant numbers of individuals will die in the pool waiting for a transplant. Three things can be done to avoid this: (1) medical criteria can be made stricter, perhaps by adding a more rigorous notion of "quality" of life to longevity and prospects for rehabilitation; (2) resources devoted to transplantation and organ procurement can be increased; or (3) individuals can be persuaded not to attempt to join the pool.

Of these three options, only the third has the promise of both conserving resources and promoting autonomy. While most persons medically eligible for a transplant would probably want one, some would not—at least if they understood all that was involved, including the need for a lifetime commitment to daily immunosuppression medications, and periodic medical monitoring for rejection symptoms. Accordingly, it makes public policy sense to publicize the risks and side effects of transplantation, and to require careful explanations of the procedure be given to prospective patients *before* they undergo medical screening. It is likely that by the time patients come to the transplant center they have made up their minds and would do almost anything to get the transplant. Nonetheless, if there are patients who, when confronted with all the facts, would voluntarily elect not to proceed, we enhance both their own freedom and the efficiency and cost-effectiveness of the transplantation system by screening them out as early as possible.

Conclusion

Choices among patients that seem to condemn some to death and give others an opportunity to survive will always be tragic. Society has developed a number of mechanisms to make such decisions more acceptable by camouflaging them. In an era of scarce resources and conscious cost containment, such mechanisms will become public, and they will be usable only if they are fair and efficient. If they are not so perceived, we will shift from one mechanism to another in an effort to continue the illusion that tragic choices really don't have to be made, and that we can simultaneously move toward equity of access, quality of services, and cost containment without any challenges to our values. Along with the prostitute, the playboy, and the poet, we all need to be involved in the development of an access model to extreme and expensive medical technologies with which we can live.

Notes

1   Calabresi, G., Bobbitt, P. *Tragic Choices*. New York: Norton, 1978.
2   Fletcher, J. Our shameful waste of human tissue. In: Cutler, D.R. (ed): *The Religious Situation*. Boston: Beacon Press, 1969; 223–252.
3   Quoted in Fox, R., Swazey, J. *The Courage to Fail*. Chicago: Univ of Chicago Press, 1974; 232.
4   Sanders, D. & Dukeminier, J. Medical advance and legal lag: hemodialysis and kidney transplantation. *UCLA L Rev* 1968; 15:357.
5   Rettig, R.A. The policy debate on patient care financing for victims of end stage renal disease. *Law & Contemporary Problems* 1976; 40:196.
6   President's Commission for the Study of Ethical Problems in Medicine. *Securing Access to Health Care*. US Govt Printing Office, 1983; 25.
7   Annas, G.J. Ethics committees on neonatal care: substantive protection or procedural diversion? *Am J Public Health* 1984; 74:843–845.
8   Bayer, R. Justice and health care in an era of cost containment: allocating scarce medical resources. *Soc Responsibility* 1984; 9:37–52.
9   Annas, G.J. Allocation of artificial hearts in the year 2002: *Minerva v National Health Agency. Am J Law Med* 1977; 3:59–76.
10 Commentary: UK's poor record in treatment of renal failure. *Lancet* July 7, 1984; 53.
11 Evans, R. Health care technology and the inevitability of resource allocation and rationing decisions, Part II. *JAMA* 1983; 249:2208, 2217.

Ethics of Queuing for Coronary Artery Bypass Grafting in Canada

Jafna L. Cox

The primary objective of Canadian health care policy is "to facilitate reasonable access to health services without financial or other barriers."[1] However, Canada's assets are finite. Limits on health care funding have resulted in rationing by queue when fixed medical resources have not met demand. Although a policy of managed delay is preferable to one of restricted access, there are major concerns about patient safety and justice. Furthermore, rationing engenders a conflict between a physician's traditional responsibility to the individual patient and the exigencies of medical practice in the universal health care system, wherein a broader responsibility to society is required. This conflict cannot be reconciled at the bedside.

The process currently used to queue patients for coronary artery bypass grafting (CABG) in Canada provides an ideal paradigm for reviewing these issues. It follows explicit, physician-established guidelines based on medical need and includes peer review to ensure their just application. This strategy allows rational selection of patients with low vital risk and, I will argue, an ethical solution to the dilemma of competing physician responsibilities to individual patients and to society.

Limits on Access to CABG in Canada

In 1988–89, a dramatic increase in referrals for CABG in Canada overtook caseload growth.[2] Patients across the country waited a mean of 22.6 weeks for elective surgery,[3] and some died. Although government pro-

Jafna L. Cox, "Ethics of Queuing for Coronary Artery Bypass Grafting in Canada," *Canadian Medical Association Journal*, vol. 151, 949–953. © 1994. Reprinted by permission of the publisher.

vided funding to augment surgical capacity[4] a mismatch between CABG demand and supply persisted.

Canadian physicians endeavoured to obtain timely surgery for their patients. However, approaches to queuing patients were inconsistent.[4] In Toronto, interhospital differences in mean wait times were as great as eight weeks. In the hospital with the shortest queues, patients referred by offsite cardiologists waited twice as long as similar ones referred by their onsite colleagues.[5] Similarly, in British Columbia analysts noted an "impressive lack" of coordinated patient referral.[6]

Panacea of Increased Funding

Canadian physicians would prefer not to have to queue their patients. A theoretically attractive expedient is yet more spending to expand surgical facilities. But bypass surgery is costly, ranging from $10,982 to $33,676 with a mean of $14,328 in 1988 Canadian dollars,[7] and health care is only one of many competing social programs that government must finance.

Waste and poor management exist. However, more efficient management is unlikely, by itself, to obviate the need for rationing:[8] the Canadian health care system is expensive despite efficient management (administrative fees being half those in the United States[9]), yet queues persist.

More important, increased medical spending to expand services does not inevitably result in better health. Greater availability of revascularization facilities leads to increased service use despite unclear survival benefit.[10,11] Indeed, revascularization facilities and procedures in Canada are few only by comparison with those in the United States.[12]

Solution of Patient Prioritization

Canadian physicians dealt with CABG queues by developing a more efficient referral process, including a rational system of assessing patient priority. This evolved, with regional modifications, from triage guidelines published in 1990 by a consensus panel.[13] In general, patients are referred, and an urgency ranking based on explicit clinical and diagnostic criteria is requested. A conference of cardiovascular specialists uses these same guidelines to review the suitability and relative urgency of surgery among all patients referred and hence ensures appropriate order in the queue. Although the process may have improved, concerns persist about its safety and fairness.

Safety of Queuing Patients for CABG

Highly publicized anecdotal accounts of patients dying while awaiting surgery neglect the immediate and delayed risks of the procedure itself.[6] In California hundreds of excess deaths result from readily available CABG at low-volume (hence high-risk) centers, and Wikler[14] questions whether in Canada the number of excess deaths due to queuing is greater.

Appropriately applied guidelines can distinguish between patients requiring immediate care and those at lower risk.[15-17] The vital risk of a six-week wait in a patient with mild to moderate stable angina, three-vessel disease and impaired left ventricular function is approximately 0.25%.[18] This is also the average risk of death from medical negligence during hospitalization, as documented in the Harvard-New York State Medical Practice Study.[18]

Indeed, the true clinical impact of the queue is unlikely to show up as excess patient deaths or major complications.[15,16] Rather, what need to be assessed are the effects on patients of persistent symptoms and the frustration and anxiety associated with waiting, as well as the hidden social and economic costs of ongoing (often intensive) medical care, lost work days, and sick benefits.[4] Anxiety could be lessened through broader appreciation that most CABG is palliative, that the vital risk associated with waiting is consequently small, and that ongoing stable symptoms need not relate to prognosis.[19]

Justice of Queuing Patients for CABG

Although CABG queues have gained particular notoriety, access to health care has always been circumscribed.[4,20] Financial factors impede access in the United States, where some 58 million people were without medical insurance at some time in 1992.[21] In Canada, implicit nonfinancial rationing in the form of queues exists instead.[22]

There is nothing inherently wrong with rationing, especially by means of queues that delay but do not deny access altogether.[22] However, the process must be safe, fair and justifiable not simply economically but also medically and ethically.[23] The law does not proscribe selection by preset, explicit allocation criteria that are rational and nondiscriminatory.[24]

Physicians tend to allocate scarce health care resources according to medical need.[25-28] Ethicists may argue whether this is the most reasonable precept to follow, but it is legally and ethically sound if the medical judgments are defensible.[27-31] According to Sulmasy,[30] physicians may be wrong in their judgements, but unless culpably ignorant they cannot be held to be acting unjustly. To ensure procedural justice and hence equal treatment of similar patients, guidelines should preferably be set and administered at higher levels of social organization (e.g., by a committee of peers).[29-31] The efficacy of a given therapy for a given patient is another morally relevant criterion.[32] The appropriate balance of urgency (patient need) and efficacy (likelihood of therapeutic success) is a critical issue for any allocation system.

When medical utility and the probability of success are roughly equal among candidates, rationing systems generally use length of wait as the fairest way to make the final selection.[33] Although imperfect, this rule of "first come, first served" has legal and ethical sanction.[31,34,35] Criticism that the process does not compensate for such impediments as distance from and ease of travel to a medical centre, which might influence one's position on the queue,[36] is less compelling in Canada, where regionalization of cardiovascular surgical services minimizes such potential inequities in access.

Principles of medical utility and of "first come, first served" are used to build the CABG queue in Canada. All medically deserving patients are considered equally, but the sickest—for whom the procedure can make the greatest difference—receive precedence.

Challenges to Queuing for CABG

Most commonly, challenges to queuing arise from patients or their physicians seeking shorter wait times. Patients have sought to jump the queue on the basis of personal connections, professional courtesy, and social merit, the latter having been proposed as a possible criterion for allocating scarce resources.[31] However, decisions based on social merit are difficult to justify given the lack of an acceptable method for assessing relative social worth. By arbitrarily prolonging the anxiety and frustration of patients passed over as well as increasing the risk associated with extended waiting, queue jumping on the basis of personal connections or professional courtesy is indefensible.

Some argue that by providing patients with therapy at different times queuing is unfair. An egalitarian theory of justice in the distribution of health care has been proposed by Rawls[37] and by Young[35] and Daniels.[36] In its most radical form, this theory holds that any deviation from absolute equality in distribution, including differences in wait time for therapy, is unjust. However, Kluge[38] offers a compelling rebuttal that emphasizes "equity rather than equality," since the provision of equal health care services to patients with unequal needs only perpetuates an unjustified inequity. Furthermore, the Canada Health Act promises "reasonable" and not "equal" access.

A different challenge comes from those willing to pay for prompt surgery. Libertarians argue that economic and social benefits should be allotted in proportion to a person's contribution to those benefits, and they support the distribution of health care services according to ability to pay.[26,39] However, this view runs counter to Canadian health care policy, which strives to eliminate financial barriers in access to health care.[1,22,40] Recent work suggests that the ability to pay led to queue jumping and hence unjust access to heart and liver transplantation in the United States in the late 1980s.[41]

Ultimately, the challenge to queuing comes from patients' demands for a right to specific and prompt treatment or from demands by physicians for a right to manage patients how and when they see fit. These individual rights may conflict with the rights of other individuals needing medical care, with the professionals involved in distributing that care or with society as a whole.[25] Indeed, to the extent that maximizing the care of an individual either restricts the resources available to others or drives up costs for others, there will be a conflict between that individual and society, which is itself a collection of individuals with their own perceived rights.[42] Comparative justice demands a fair share, not an excessive one.[26] Physicians invoking a right to manage patients as they see fit are faced with David Eddy's[43] question: "Who gave physicians that right?"

Ethical Dilemma: Physicians and Queuing

Physicians in a universal health care system face an ethical dilemma arising out of conflicting responsibilities to the individual patient and to society. A fiduciary relationship compels physicians to advocate on behalf of their patients, and many clinicians consider unethical any intrusion of economic considerations. However, whether costs are interpreted as a financial or other kind of sacrifice, the investment of resources on one patient comes at the expense of another. To ignore this cost imposed on another individual is itself unethical.[44] Moreover, competition between individual physicians advocating on behalf of individual patients in a constrained health care system can be detrimental, as highlighted by the discrepant referral practices that exacerbated the CABG crisis in the late 1980s.

Analogous to the traditional doctor-patient relationship, there is a public health model under which physicians have obligations to people who are not their patients.[28] Moreover, physicians cannot simultaneously be advocates of their patients and also serve as financial guardians of society without incurring divided loyalties and ethical peril.[28,30,35,45]

Indeed, the traditional ethic of the physician's responsibility to the patient cannot be adequately reconciled with the countervailing demands of social justice in a health care system promising universal access to limited resources. Hence, the conference of specialists is important as a gatekeeper, a forum for debating which priority should prevail. When physicians disagree in matters of clinical judgment but agree on the principle of mobilizing resources for the good of each patient according to need, unequal treatment of similar patients may occur without injustice.[27,28] This does not imply that choosing one patient over another should be easy or free from guilt. However, peer review permits impartial assessment and broader opinion, and it safeguards equal treatment of similar patients; at the same time more efficient patient processing results in decreased illness and death among those on waiting lists. Consensus judgment additionally provides a legal defence for triage decisions.

The health care system in Canada has promised its consumers reasonable access to all appropriate services. As stakeholders, physicians should work in concert with their colleagues to uphold that ideal. This does not imply that physicians should become agents of public or economic policy with cost-effectiveness as the only relevant consideration. Rather, they should continue to design guidelines for the just distribution of scarce health care resources, since it is through the efficient and effective management of medical services that benefits to both the individual and society can be maximized.

Because any universal system must allow for variation in individual perceptions of need, in that different values are placed on each disability or condition, physicians must remain patients' advocates. They can thereby ensure that guidelines are relevant to the specific needs of patients and, moreover, that such guidelines have been fairly applied. Appropriate physician advocacy on behalf of patients, together with a committee of physicians acting as gatekeepers in accordance with explicit guidelines, will provide an ethical mechanism for balancing competing claims to limited resources. Thus, within the constraints on health resource availability physicians remain free to promote the interests of their patients. At the same time, consensus guidelines and peer review, through the committee, protect the interests of society by imposing reasonable limits on what might be done and when. Although this represents some loss of physician autonomy over the management of the individual patient there is a corresponding broadening of responsibility toward society.[43]

Finally, as much as they must restrain demagogic attitudes and inflammatory responses to allocation problems, physicians should avoid the trap of becoming silent queue managers. Queuing can be performed fairly and at low risk given an adequate level of medical services. There is a danger, however, that government may withhold the funds needed to maintain or expand such services on the mistaken assumption that current triage efforts will continue to be effective. Physicians and their patients must determine how much of a given medical service is adequate in terms of minimizing patient risk and discomfort; guidelines should be modified accordingly. They are duty bound to speak up when resources are so restricted that queues put patients at risk or make their discomfort intolerable.

Conclusion

Queues provide an imperfect but practical solution whenever fixed resources cannot meet demand. They are defensible if considered a temporary delay in the delivery of a service and if there is no significant adverse effect on patient health. Indeed, a policy of managed delay has advantages over systems of financial rationing, which may deny access altogether. Rationing decisions are difficult, but queuing is ethical if based on medical need and if patients understand the process, its rationale and the low associated risk. Competing responsibilities to patients and society may present physicians with an ethical dilemma. However, although their primary obligation is to their patients, their collective responsibility is to establish and follow guidelines that ensure an appropriate level of care as well as efficient and equitable allocation of available resources. Since increased funding is doubtful, physician cooperation in the rational distribution of scarce health commodities will be needed to preserve the ideal of a universal health care system. Nevertheless, rather than simply manage queues physicians must remain vigilant against cuts in medical services that would unacceptably put patients at risk.

Notes

I am indebted to Dr. C. David Naylor and Professor Arthur Schafer for reviewing the manuscript and providing helpful comments. However, the views expressed are mine, and responsibility for them rests solely with me.

1   *Canada Health Act*, RSC 1985, c6, s3.

2   Ugnat, A.M., Naylor, C.D. Trends in coronary artery bypass grafting in Ontario from 1981 to 1989. *Can Med Assoc J* 1993; 148: 569–575.

3   Higginson, L.A.J., Cairns, J.A., Keon, W.J. et al. Rates of cardiac catheterization, coronary angioplasty and open-heart surgery in adults in Canada. *Can Med Assoc J* 1992; 146: 921–925.

4   Naylor, C.D. A different view of queues in Ontario. *Health Aff (Millwood)* 1991; 10: 110–128.

5   Naylor, C.D., Levinton, C.M., Wheeler, S.M. et al. Queuing for coronary surgery during severe supply–demand mismatch in a Canadian referral centre: a case study of implicit rationing. *Soc Sci Med* 1993; 37(1): 61–67.

6   Katz, S.I., Mizgala, H.F., Welch, G. British Columbia sends patients to Seattle for coronary artery surgery: bypassing the queue in Canada. *JAMA* 1991; 266: 1108–1111.

7   Krueger, H., Goncalves, J.L., Caruth, F.M. et al. Coronary artery bypass grafting: How much does it cost? *Can Med Assoc J* 1992; 146: 163–168.

8   Brook, R.H., Lohr, K.N.G. Will we need to ration effective health care? *Issues Sci Technol* 1986; 3: 68–77.

9   Woolhandler, S., Himmelstein, D.U. The deteriorating administrative efficiency of the US health care system. *N Engl J Med* 1991; 324: 1253–1258.

10 Every, N.R., Larson, E.B., Litwin, P.E. et al. The association between on-site cardiac catheterization facilities and the use of coronary angiography after acute myocardial infarction. *N Engl J Med* 1993; 329: 546–551.

11 Cox, J.L., Chen, C., Naylor, C.D. Revascularization after acute myocardial infarction: Impact of hospital teaching status and on-site invasive facilities. *J Gen Int Med* 1994.

12 Collins-Nakai, R.L., Huysmans, H.A., Scully, H.E. Access to cardiovascular care: an international comparison. *J Am Coll Cardiol* 1992; 19: 1477–1485.

13 Naylor, C.D., Baigrie, R.S., Goldman, B.S. et al. Revascularisation Panel and Consensus Methods Group: Assessment of priority for coronary revascularisation procedures. *Lancet* 1990; 335: 1070–1073.

14 Wikler, D. Ethics and rationing: "Whether", "how", or "how much"? *J Am Geriatr Soc* 1992; 40: 398–403.

15 Cox, J.L., Petrie, J.F., Pollak, P.T. et al. Is queuing for coronary artery bypass surgery safe? A Canadian perspective. [abstract] *Circulation* 1993; 88(4 pt 2): I-10.

16 Naylor, G.D., Morgan, C.D., Levinton, C.M. et al. Waiting for coronary revascularization in Toronto: 2 years' experience with a regional referral office. *Can Med Assoc J* 1993; 149: 955–962.

17 Morris, A.L., Roos, L.L., Brazauskas, R. et al. Managing scarce services: a waiting list approach to cardiac catheterization. *Med Care* 1990; 28: 784–792.

18 Rachlis, M.M., Olak, J., Naylor, C.D. The vital risk of delayed coronary surgery: lessons from the randomized trials. *Iatrogenics* 1991; 1: 103–111.

19 Cox, J., Naylor, C.D. The Canadian Cardiovascular Society grading scale for angina of effort: Is it time for refinements? *Ann Intern Med* 1992; 117: 677–683.

20 Blank, R.H. Rationing medicine: hard choices in the 1990s. *Am J Gastroenterol* 1992; 87: 1076–1084.

21 Swartz, K. Dynamics of people without health insurance: Don't let the numbers fool you. *JAMA* 1994; 271: 64–66.

22 Naylor, C.D. The Canadian health care system: A model for America to emulate? *Health Economics* 1992; 1: 19–37.

23 Relman, A.S. The trouble with rationing. *N Engl J Med* 1990; 323: 911–913.

24 Sanders, D., Jesse, D. Jr. Medical advance and legal lag. Hemodialysis and kidney transplantation. *UCLA Law Review* 1968; 15: 366–380.

25 Horvath, D.G. The ethics of resource allocation. *Med J Aust* 1990; 153: 437–438.

26 Beauchamp, T.L., Childress, J.F. *Principles of Biomedical Ethics,* 3rd ed, Oxford University Press, New York, 1989: 256–306.

27 Ashley, B.M., O'Rourke, K.D. *Health Care Ethics: a Theological Analysis,* Catholic Association of the United States, St Louis, Mo, 1982: 239–242.

28 Macklin, R. *Mortal Choices: Ethical Dilemmas in Modern Medicine,* Houghton Mifflin Company, Boston, 1987: 149–181.

29 Edwards, R.B., Graber, G.C. *Bio-Ethics,* Harcourt Brace Jovanovich, Publishers, San Diego, 1988: 699–713.

30 Sulmasy, D.P. Physicians, cost control, and ethics. *Ann Intern Med* 1992; 116: 920–926.

31 Rescher, N. The allocation of exotic medical lifesaving therapy. *Ethics* 1969; 79: 173–186.

32 Kilner, J.F. *Who Lives? Who Dies? Ethical Criteria and Patient Selection.* Yale University Press, New Haven, Conn, 1990.

33 Task Force on Organ Transplantation: *Organ Transplantation: Issues and Recommendations,* US Department of Health and Human Services, Apr 1986.

34 Childress, J.F. Who shall live when not all can live? *Soundings* 1970; 53: 339–355.

35 Young, R. Some criteria for making decisions concerning the distribution of scarce medical resources. *Theory and Decision* 1975; 6: 439–455.

36 Daniels, N. *Just Health Care,* Cambridge University Press, Cambridge, England, 1985.

37 Rawls, J. *A Theory of Justice,* Harvard University Press, Cambridge, Mass, 1971.

38 Kluge, E.-H.W. *Biomedical Ethics in a Canadian Context,* Prentice-Hall, Scarborough, Ont, 1992: 206–235.

39 Sade, R.M. Medical care as a right: a refutation. *N Engl J Med* 1971; 285: 1288–1292.

40 Evans, R.G. The real issues. *J Health Polit Policy Law* 1992; 17: 739–762.

41 Ozminkowski, R.J., Friedman, B., Taylor, Z. Access to heart and liver transplantation in the late 1980s. *Med Care* 1993; 31: 1027–1042.

42 Eddy, D.M. The individual vs society: Is there a conflict? *JAMA* 1991; 265: 1446, 1449–1450.

43 Eddy, D.M. Broadening the responsibilities of practitioners: the team approach. *JAMA* 1993; 269: 1849–1855.

44 Williams, A. Cost-effectiveness analysis: Is it ethical? *J Med Ethics* 1992; 18: 7–11.

45 Pellegrino, E.D. Rationing health care: the ethics of medical gatekeeping. *J Contemp Health Law Policy* 1986; 2: 23–45.

Rationing in Practice:
The Case of In Vitro Fertilization
Sharon Redmayne and Rudolf Klein

Explicit decisions by purchasers to stop offering specific forms of treatment, on the Oregon model,[1] are still very much the exception in the National Health Service. For the most part rationing takes the traditional, less visible, form of limiting the resources that are available for particular services and leaving it to doctors to determine priorities between different procedures and patients. There are, however, exceptions. One such is in vitro fertilization. Analysis of 114 purchasing plans for 1992–93 found six authorities which explicitly stated that they would not be buying any in vitro fertilization or gamete intrafallopian transfer treatment for their populations.[2] At the same time, other purchasers were continuing to buy in vitro fertilization and, some were even planning to put extra money into the service.

The case of in vitro fertilization therefore provides an intriguing, and rare, opportunity to explore the way in which such explicit rationing decisions are reached. In vitro fertilization produces results, although there is some debate about its success rate and about the circumstances in which its use is appropriate.[3] In contrast to procedures like tattoo removal (struck off the National Health Service menu by seven purchasing authorities), it cannot be seen as a response to a self-inflicted injury or as a tribute to vanity. Furthermore, the use of in vitro fertilization is widespread in Europe: in France its use is reimbursed by the social security system, and in Belgium, Denmark, and Norway the state will bear most or all of the cost.[4]

Why, then, do purchasers disagree about the desirability of buying this procedure? What evidence and arguments were used in coming to these

Sharon Redmayne and Rudolf Klein, "Rationing in Practice: The Case of In Vitro Fertilization," from *BMJ* (*British Medical Journal*), vol. 306, 1521–1524. © 1993 by BMJ Publishing Group. Reprinted by permission of the publisher.

decisions? What local circumstances or pressures influenced the decision to buy or not to buy? And can any general insights into the dilemmas and problems of rationing be derived from this specific case?

To answer these questions, we compare three purchasing authorities which decided not to buy in vitro fertilization with three others which took the opposite decision. In each case our account is based on the documents produced by the authorities and informed by the views of relevant health authority officials, who were either interviewed or contacted by letter. These are in no sense a sample. Apart from anything else, we do not know how many purchasers have quietly decided not to offer in vitro fertilization without making their views explicit. All six authorities are gainers, if to differing degrees, under the weighted capitation formula. The differences between them cannot therefore be explained by variations in resource constraints.

Nonpurchasers of In Vitro Fertilization

Health Authority A

This first health authority provides a subfertility service but not in vitro fertilization or gamete intrafallopian transfer. The scope of the infertility service was one of the issues discussed at the authority's "choices for health day," which brought together a range of interested professionals to rank a list of bids for development money. They decided that in vitro fertilization would not be offered because of its cost: the health authority, it was argued, should not spend so much money on people who were not "ill." The view was not unanimous: the women were generally more sympathetic to the case for in vitro fertilization than the men. They argued that the mental distress of being infertile should be taken into account and that the people of the district should have the choice available to them.

The health authority decided that while people on the waiting list for in vitro fertilization in 1992–93 should still be seen the treatment would thereafter be provided only as an extra contractual referral. In practice, however the authority has been turning down such extracontractual referrals. Several factors have influenced the authority in this stance, quite apart from the views of the "choices for health day" meeting. The general practitioners are happy with current service provision and are not exerting any pressure to extend it. Neighboring health authorities do not provide in vitro fertilization either. There is also a general feeling that, since the district is relatively affluent, people can afford to be treated privately.

Health Authority B

As part of its assisted conception services the second health authority provides donor insemination and intrauterine insemination but no in vitro fertilization or gamete intrafallopian transfer. It has deliberately decided against purchasing in vitro fertilization because of cost. The nearest provider unit charges about £2,000 per cycle. In contrast, donor insemination costs £70 per cycle. Instead of buying in vitro fertilization, the authority has therefore decided to strengthen its donor insemination services. Requests for in vitro fertilization under the extra contractual referral procedure are turned down.

The authority's reasoning is that equity demands that any service provided should give everyone requiring treatment a fair chance of getting it. To buy only a few cycles of in vitro fertilization is therefore unfair. Also, the authority does not consider that in vitro fertilization represents good value for money. Although the success rate of in vitro fertilization is actually better than for donor insemination in terms of babies produced, the cost per birth is higher. Moreover, for every cycle of in vitro fertilization, which has a one in four chance of success, a new hip can be bought.

So far, the authority's decision about in vitro fertilization has brought no backlash from the local community. There does not appear to be either a community or a professional lobby pressing for the purchase of in vitro fertilization. If there were a groundswell of opinion the authority would reconsider its position.

Authority C

Authority C differs from the previous two in that it did not decide explicitly against providing in vitro fertilization but simply gave it a low priority. It was originally included in the list of purchasing developments for 1992–93, but it was not high enough on the list of priorities to justify additional funds. In vitro fertilization is thus excluded from the authority's contracts, although it can be made available through extra contractual referrals. In effect in vitro fertilization has become a casualty of the competitive battle for resources.

Not surprisingly, given this decision-making process, there has been no extensive discussion or assessment of in vitro fertilization in this district. The authority has largely drawn on the results of national research and appears to have been strongly influenced by the director of public health's view that the clinical effectiveness of in vitro fertilization treatment is generally low.

Purchasers of In Vitro Fertilization

Authority D

Authority D decided to buy in vitro fertilization as part of a whole range of fertility services. It calculated that it would cost £280,000 per year to provide subfertility treatment for all the residents who might present, but it could afford to put only £150,000 into the service. So it decided to fund 20 in vitro fertilization cycles, agreeing with the providers on the criteria to be used in choosing the beneficiaries. It also agreed with the provider on the number of embryos to be used in order to limit the number of multiple births and the pressure on maternity services.

Local circumstances clearly influenced this decision. A local provider of in vitro fertilization is already in place, and the unit is highly regarded and has strong support among clinicians. The consultant in charge of the infertility service is also an effective lobbyist.

Members of the authority played an active role in the decision, examining the evidence about the extent of infertility problems in the community and the medical evidence about the effectiveness of in vitro fertilization. Four considerations appear to have determined their views.

First, they concluded that infertility can cause psychological harm as well as marital difficulties. Second, they attached much importance to the role of the family. Third, they saw themselves as having a moral obligation to put more money into their subfertility package for in vitro fertilization since, at the other end of the scale, they purchase abortions, sterilisations, and contraception services. To spend additional money preventing babies being born without also doing likewise to help the infertile was felt to be ethically unjustifiable. Fourth, they believed that it would breach the National Health Service's principle of equality of access to deny in vitro fertilization treatment of local women when it is available in other districts.

Authority E came into being only in April 1993, as the result of the amalgamation of three districts, and decided to purchase about 62 cycles of in vitro fertilization in 1993–94. There are 24 in vitro fertilization centers within acceptable traveling distance, whose costs range from £498 to £2,546, excluding drugs, so the authority is inviting tenders from these providers. Each center has been asked to supply information on outcomes, numbers of treatment cycles, and patient selection to help the authority in choosing the most cost effective options.

This authority's decision reflects its view that subfertility is a health care problem with very definite physiological, psychological, and social implications. It also differs from the decisions made by other authorities in that it was based on an elaborate needs assessment exercise carried out by the public health department.

The report that emerged from this exercise integrated epidemiological evidence, the results of a survey of consultants in obstetrics and gynecology, and information from local in vitro fertilization centers. It estimated, on the basis of a survey of the evidence by the *Effective Health Care Bulletin*,[3] that about 333 women a year would need in vitro fertilization or gamete intrafallopian transfer but recommended that only in vitro fertilization should be bought. The report argued that gamete intrafallopian transfer did not have in vitro fertilization's advantage of detecting poor fertilization and bypassing tubal damage.

The authority subsequently carried out a survey of consultants to establish local need and decided to buy 62 cycles of in vitro fertilization. This still left the question of how those limited resources should be allocated—for example, what rationing principles should be used. Here the decision has been to use two criteria: age and family size. Women over 40 will be excluded because the success of in vitro fertilization decreases with age, and only couples who have no children or only one child will be considered. The final selection will be made by the consultant in charge, and there will be a maximum of two cycles per patient. In addition, purchasers and providers are to produce shared protocols for general practitioners, consultants, and the specialist centres to improve the investigation and treatment of subfertility.

Authority F

The last authority decided to fund in vitro fertilization and gamete intra-fallopian transfer for the first time ever in 1993–94, although it has not yet fixed the budgetary allocation. Previously it had refused to provide funding because of doubts about effectiveness in the early pioneering years, concern about possible side effects, and the belief that the treatments, as new technologies, should be developed and tested more centrally.

The decision to change policy reflects the influence of two factors. First, local pressure groups have been vociferous in pressing the authority to fund in vitro fertilization and gamete intrafallopian transfer. Second, a policy review carried out by the authority's public health departments dispelled some of the earlier doubts about effectiveness.

The policy review estimated that about 270 couples a year would require subfertility services, of whom some 50 might benefit from in vitro fertilization. It also recognised, however, that the high Asian population in the area may make the demand on the service greater. As in authority E, demand is therefore likely to exceed supply, thus raising, once again, the question of selection. No formal criteria for in vitro fertilization treatment have yet been laid down. But current discussions suggest that criteria for selection are likely to include primary versus secondary infertility, and prognosis. In addition, a local protocol for managing subfertility has been developed with general practitioners and obstetricians in the hope that this will save money by reducing unnecessary and repeated investigations.

The Dynamics of Rationing

Our six cameo case studies do not purport to illustrate the whole range of decision making among purchasers. But they do identify some of the main issues. First, they suggest the importance of local champions for any given service or procedure. In vitro fertilization is more likely to be purchased in those authorities where there is a local provider and, thus, a local constituency of support. Pressure from general practitioners and the community is another factor that influences purchasing authorities. Such influence may work both positively and negatively: if there is no pressure authorities may conclude that there is no demand.

Second, the case studies also indicate the importance of public health departments, both as the interpreters of the evidence about effectiveness and value for money and as assessors of need.

Third, however, the case studies show some differences of opinion about what should count as a need when it comes to allocating resources—for example, where the frontiers of the National Health Service's responsibilities should be drawn. This issue is also raised by decisions not to buy various cosmetic procedures. Thus authority A was not prepared to spend money on individuals who were not perceived to be really "ill." In contrast, the purchasers of in vitro fertilization believed that there was a health need which had to be addressed. They were convinced by the arguments of the Royal College of Obstetricians and Gynaecologists[5] and others[6] that the inability to have children can cause psychological distress and damage— that the "pain of childlessness is every bit as great as that of osteoarthritis of the hip."[7]

Effectiveness

Fourth, those authorities which accept that infertility does represent a legitimate claim on National Health Service resources then had to ask whether in vitro fertilization was the best way of meeting that need. In considering this question the authorities had to address questions of effectiveness. A recent *Effective Health Care Bulletin* on the management of subfertility concluded that techniques such as in vitro fertilization are quite effective, although this is often offset by poor organisation of the service.[3] Success rates have increased over the past few years,[8] and one study concluded that in couples where the woman was under 40 and the man had normal sperm a pregnancy rate of 30% per cycle had been achieved by 1991.[9]

Fifth, however, showing that a treatment is effective—in the sense of producing results—does not necessarily demonstrate that it should be purchased. Inevitably such decisions merge with questions of value for money, and this involves comparison with other claims on resources. Questions also arise about whether such comparisons should be made solely in terms of the relative cost-effectiveness of different treatments within the same field (in vitro fertilization or donor insemination?) or whether they should be made between treatments in different fields (in vitro fertilization or hips?). Whichever sort of comparison is done it seems to demand a rough and ready assessment of the relative health gains produced by different interventions. The case studies suggest that authorities do not make such systematic comparisons—no doubt because the required information is not available. Quality adjusted life years–style analyses were conspicuous by their absence.

Sixth, the case studies illustrate two quite different types of rationing decisions. On the one hand, there are decisions about how much to allocate to a particular type of activity. On the other hand, having decided to support a particular type of activity an authority then has to decide who to treat when supply falls short of demand. Even authorities which are buying in vitro fertilization have to make the second type of decision. Interestingly, too, the case studies suggest that—in the case of in vitro fertilization at least—authorities are beginning to become involved in devising criteria and protocols for allocating treatment to individual patients. This trend can be expected to become more general.

Equity

Last, the case studies raise some fundamental questions for the National Health Service. Does the principle of equity of access require that everyone should have an equal chance of treatment irrespective of where he or she lives? Both authority B and authority D assumed that it did, though they drew diametrically opposed conclusions. And if equity does demand an equal chance of treatment (at least once a treatment has passed the experimental stage) does this mean, in turn, that rationing decisions should be made nationally, since it cannot be left to individual purchasers to determine what services should or should not be available? Again, in determining priorities, how legitimate is it for health authorities to take into account the availability of services in the private sector? Does not the fact that an estimated 90% of births achieved through in vitro fertilization in the United Kingdom (though not all in United Kingdom nationals) are the result of private treatment[10] offend against the principle of equity? And if so, are we not once again left with the uncomfortable conclusion that equity demands that a service should be provided either universally— at least in the sense of giving everyone the same statistical chance of access—or not at all?

These questions, to which the answers are far from self evident, are prompted by the case of in vitro fertilization. They demonstrate, however, that the issues raised by in vitro fertilization range far beyond this particular treatment and need to be addressed in the context of the National Health Service as a whole.

Notes

The research on which this essay draws is funded by the Nuffield Provincial Hospitals Trust.

1   Klein, R. Warning signals from Oregon. *BMJ* 1992; 304:1457–8.

2   Klein, R., Redmayne, S. *Patterns of priorities.* Birmingham: NAHAT, 1992.

3   *The management of subfertility.* Leeds: School of Public Health, Leeds University, 1992 (*Effective Health Care Bulletin* No 3).

4   Gunning, J. *Human IVF, embryo research, fetal tissue for research and treatment, and abortion: international information.* London: HMSO, 1990.

5   Fertility Committee, Royal College of Obstetricians and Gynaecologists. *Infertility: guidelines for practice.* London: RCOG Press, 1992.

6   Mazor, M.D. Emotional reactions to infertility. In: Mazor, M.D., Simons, H.F., eds. *Infertility: medical, emotional, and social considerations.* New York: Human Sciences Press Inc, 1984:29–39.

7   Pain of childlessness. *BMJ* 1991;302:1345.

8   Human Fertilisation and Embryology Authority. *Annual report.* London: HMSO, 1992.

9   Hull, M.G.R., Eddowes, H.A., Fahy, U., Abuzeid, M.I., Mills, M.S., Cahill, D.J. et al. Expectations of assisted conception for infertility. *BMJ* 1992;304:1465–9.

10 Hunt, L. Infertility units face struggle for survival. *Independent*, 1992; 2 Nov:4, cols 1–7.

PART III

International Perspectives and Emerging Issues

Reforming the Health Care System:
The Universal Dilemma
Uwe E. Reinhardt

Introduction

The human condition surrounding the delivery of health care is the same everywhere in the world: the providers of health care seek to give their patients the maximum feasible degree of physical relief, but they also aspire to a healthy slice of the gross national product (GNP) as a reward for their efforts. Patients seek from health care providers the maximum feasible degree of physical relief, but, collectively, they also seek to minimize the slice of the GNP that they must cede to providers as the price for that care.

In other words, while there typically is a meeting of the minds between patients and providers on the *clinical* side of the health care transaction, there very often is conflict on the *economic* front. It has always been so, since time immemorial, and it will always be so. It is part of the human condition. Health insurance does not lessen this perennial economic conflict; it merely transfers it from the patient's bedside to the desk of some private or public bureaucrat who is charged with guarding a collective insurance treasury.

However, health insurance does realign the parties to the economic fray. Because insurance shields patients from the cost of their medical treatments at the point of service, it tends to move them squarely into the providers' corner when they are sick. Usually, in that corner, patients rail, with little chance of success, against the heartless bureaucrats who refuse to finance procedures. On the other hand, when patients are healthy

Uwe E. Reinhardt, "Reforming the Health Care System: The Universal Dilemma," from *American Journal of Law and Medicine*, vol. 19, 21–36. © 1993 by Uwe E. Reinhardt and *American Journal of Law and Medicine*. Reprinted by permission of the publisher and the author.

and faced with mounting taxes or insurance premiums, they are typically found in the bureaucrats' corner. In that corner, patients rail against health care providers' voracious financial appetite and holler for cost controls.

In this essay, I explore how different nations approach the universal twin problems of modern health care: the provisions of access to health care on equitable terms and the control of health care costs. It is true that there is a rich variety of alternative approaches to these twin problems. It is also true that virtually every developed nation is now dissatisfied with its health care system and seeks to reform it. Unfortunately, there does not seem to be a single *ideal* solution.

Controlling the Transfer of GNP to Providers

Society can control the total annual transfer of GNP to health care providers through the demand side of the health care market, the supply side, or both. Nations differ substantially in the mix of approaches they use. Their choice of cost-control policies hinges crucially on the social role that they ascribe to health care. The two extremes of the spectrum of views on this issue are:

1. Health care is essentially a *private consumption good*, whose financing is the responsibility of its individual recipient.
2. Health care is a *social good* that should be collectively financed and available to all citizens who need health care, regardless of the individual recipient's ability to pay for that care.

Canadians and Europeans have long since reached a broad social consensus that health care is a social good. Although their health systems exhibit distinct, national idiosyncrasies, they share an obedience to that overarching, ethical precept.

Americans have never been able to reach a similarly broad political consensus regarding the point at which they would like their health care system to sit on the ideological spectrum that is defined by these two extreme views. Instead, American health policy has meandered back and forth between the two views, in step with the ideological temper of the time. During the 1960s and 1970s, the American health care system moved toward the social good end of the spectrum. On the other hand, during the 1980s, a concerted effort was made to move the system in the opposite direction. This meandering between distinct, ethical precepts has

Table 1. Alternative Mixes of Health Insurance and Health Care Delivery

	Collectivized (Socialized) Financing of Health Care			
		Private Health Insurance[a]		Direct Financing
Production and delivery	Government-financed insurance	Within a statutory framework	Within an unregulated market	Out-of-pocket by patients at point of service
Purely government-owned	A	D	G	J
Private not-for-profit entities	B	E	H	K
Private for-profit entities	C	F	I	L
	The Canadian health system	The West German health system	The private portion of the American system	

[a] Note: Technically, whenever the receipt of health care is paid for by a third party rather than the recipient at point of service, it is financed out of a *collective* pool and is, thus, "socialized" financing. In this sense, private health insurance is just as "collectivist" or "socialized" as government-provided health insurance. Both forms of financing destroy the normal workings of a market because both eliminate the individual benefit-cost calculus that is the *sine qua non* of a proper market.

produced contradictions between professed principles and actual practice that confuse and frustrate even the initiated in the United States.

Table 1 presents a menu of alternative approaches to financing and organizing health care. It makes explicit distinctions between the ownership of the health insurance mechanism and the production of health care. Almost all health care systems in the world fit into this grid, and most extend over more than one cell in the grid.

For example, the health systems of the United Kingdom and Sweden occupy primarily cell A in table 1, though private medical practices in the United Kingdom occupy cell C. One may think of cell A as socialized medicine in its purest sense because the production of health care is substantially owned by the government. Clearly, the health care system of the United States Department of Veterans Affairs also resides in cell A, as does the bulk of the health care system for the United States armed forces.

The Canadian health care system occupies primarily cells A, B, and C, as does the American federal Medicare program and the federal-state Medicaid program. Systems falling into cells A, B, and C represent *government-*

run health insurance, not *socialized medicine*, because the delivery system is largely in private hands. This distinction between *socialized insurance* and *socialized medicine* is often lost on American critics of foreign health care systems.

Germany's health care system is best described by cells D, E, and F. Health insurance in Germany is provided by a structured system of not-for-profit sickness funds that are privately administered, albeit within a federal statute that tightly regulates their conduct.[1] This statutory health insurance system has evolved gradually over the span of 100 years and now covers 88% of the population.[2] The remainder is covered by private, commercial insurers more akin to commercial insurers in the United States.[3] On the other hand, Germany's health care delivery system is a mixture of private and public, for-profit and not-for-profit, providers that is similar to the mix of providers found in the United States. In other words, the German health care system also does not represent socialized medicine, but socialized insurance.

As noted above, parts of the American health system fall squarely into cell A. Others fall into cells A, B, and C. Together, cells A through C accounted for about 44% of national health care spending in 1991.[4] The rest of the system, its private sector, is spread from cells G to L. As part of the impending reform of the American health care system, this private sector is likely to slide toward either cells D, E, and F, or even toward cells A, B, and C. The concept of "managed competition," for example, fits into cells D, E, and F, as would an "all-payer" system, under which multiple private insurance carriers would be subject to common fee schedules. On the other hand, if Congress legislated a single-payer system based on the Canadian model—or "Medicare for All"—the American system would rest in cells A, B, and C.

The Approaches Used in Canada and Europe

As noted, Canadians and Europeans typically view health care as a social good. In these countries, it is anathema to link an individual household's health care financing contribution to the health status of that household's members. Health care in these countries is collectively financed, with taxes or premiums based on the individual household's ability to pay.[5] Only a small, well-to-do minority—so far, less than 10% of the population—opts out of collective social insurance in favor of privately insured or privately financed health care.[6] Nevertheless, nearly 90% of the population typically shares one common level of quality and amenities in health care.

Control of health care costs in these countries is exercised partly by controlling the physical capacity of the supply side. The chief instrument for this purpose is formal regional health planning.[7] Planning enables policy makers to limit the number of hospital beds, big-ticket technology (such as CT scanners or lithotripters), and sometimes even the number of physicians who are issued billing numbers under these nations' health insurance systems.

However, regulatory limits on the capacity of the health care system inevitably create monopolies on the supply side. To make sure that these artificially created monopolies do not exploit their economic power, these countries generally couple health planning on the supply side with stiff price and budgetary controls imposed on the demand side. Sometimes, price controls alone are deemed sufficient to control overall health spending. However, where the intent of price controls has been thwarted through rapid increases in the volume of health services rendered, these countries have imposed strictly limited global budgets on the health care systems as a whole, or upon particular segments (e.g., hospitals and doctors). Canada, for example, has long compensated its hospitals through preset global budgets. Similarly, West Germany now operates strict, statewide expenditure caps for all physicians who practice within a state under the nation's Statutory Health Insurance system. The United Kingdom and the Nordic countries budget virtually their entire health systems.[8]

To implement their price and budget controls, Canada and the European countries tend to structure their health insurance systems so that money flows from third-party payers to health care providers through only one or a few large moneypipes. The "money pipe" throughput is then controlled through formal negotiations between regional or national associations of third-party payers and associations of providers. The negotiated prices in these countries are usually binding on providers, who may not bill patients for extra charges above these prices. Although France permits extra billing within limits, most of these countries perceive unrestrained extra billing as a violation of the spirit of health insurance.[9]

Remarkably, and in sharp contrast with the United States, Canada and Europe typically do not look to the individual patient as an agent of cost control. Usually, there is no significant flow of money from patient to provider at the time health services are received. Instead, most of these countries provide patients with comprehensive, universal *first-dollar* coverage for a wide range of services, including drugs (Canada covers drugs only for the poor). France does have copayments at the point of service for all ambulatory care and hospital care, but not for certain high-cost illnesses.[10] Furthermore, many French patients have supplemental private insurance to cover any copayments.[11]

One should not assume that Canada and the European nations eclipse patients from cost control because these nations' health policy analysts and policy makers lack the savvy of their American colleagues. American debates on health policy tend to characterize patients as "consumers" who are expected to shop around for cost-effective health care. One suspects that Canadians and Europeans are inclined to perceive patients as, for the most part, "sick persons" who should be treated as such. Table 2 suggests why that perception may be a valid one. As table 2 illustrates, the distribution of health expenditures across a population tends to be highly skewed. In the United States, for example, only 5% of the population accounts for about half of all national health expenditures in any given year, and 10% account for about seventy percent. The distribution of health expenditures in other countries is apt to present a similar pattern.

One must wonder whether the few individuals who account for the bulk of health care expenditures in any given year can actually act like regular "consumers" who shop around for cost-effective health care. Although cost sharing by patients can be shown to have some constraining effect on utilization for mild to semiserious illness,[12] it is unlikely to play a major role in the serious cases that appear to account for the bulk of national health care expenditures.

Where price and ability to pay cannot ration health care, something else must. Usually, in Canada and Europe, that non-price rationing device is a queue for elective medical procedures. At the extreme, some high-tech medical interventions, such as renal dialysis or certain organ transplantations, are simply unavailable to particular patients if the attending physician judges the likely benefits of intervention to be low. High-tech innovations are introduced rather cautiously in these nations, and only after intensive benefit-cost analysis. Therefore, at any given time, these nations' health care systems are likely to lag behind that in the United States in the degree to which a new medical technology has been adopted.[13]

Finally, the tight control on overall outlays for health care tends to preclude the often luxurious settings in which health care is dispensed to

Table 2. Distribution of Health Expenditures for the U.S. Population, by Magnitude of Expenditures, Selected Years, 1928–1987

Percent of U.S. population ranked by expenditures	1928	1963	1970	1977	1980	1987
Top 1 percent	—	17%	26%	27%	29%	30%
Top 2 percent	—	—	35	38	39	41
Top 5 percent	52%	43	50	55	55	58
Top 10 percent	—	59	66	70	70	72
Top 30 percent	93	—	88	90	90	91
Top 50 percent	—	95	96	97	96	97
Bottom 50 percent	—	5	4	3	4	3

Source: Marc L. Berk and Alan C. Monheit, *Data Watch: The Concentration of Health Expenditures: An Update*, HEALTH AFF., Winter 1992, at 145, 146.

well-insured patients in the United States. Atriums and gourmet dining in hospitals, or physician offices with plush carpets, are not common in Canada or Europe.

The Entrepreneurial American Approach

Americans have traditionally looked askance at regulation. To be sure, some regulatory controls of the supply side of health care have been attempted at various times in a number of states (e.g., through certificate-of-need laws). There have also been occasional flirtations with price controls (e.g., under Richard Nixon's presidency, or in states that regulate hospital rates).[14] For the most part, however, Americans have always viewed the supply side of their health sector as an open economic frontier in which any and all profit-seeking entrepreneurs may gain economic fortunes. Indeed, traditionally, Americans have seen the very openness of their health system to profit-seeking entrepreneurship as the main driving force that has made the American health care system, in their own eyes, the best in the world.[15]

American physicians, for example, have always prided themselves on their status as staunch "free-enterprisers," and have vigorously, although not entirely successfully, defended that status against inroads by third-party payers. Furthermore, as historian Rosemary Stevens has shown convincingly in *In Sickness and in Wealth: A History of the American Hospital in the Twentieth Century*, even the nation's so-called not-for-profit

Table 3. Cost Sharing by American Patients 1987[*]

Category of Expenditure	Mean Annual Spending per Person with that Expense	Mean Percentage of Expenditure Paid out of Pocket
All health services	$1,804	24%
All inpatient services	$7,120	8%
Inpatient physician services	$1,976	16%
Ambulatory physician services	$470	26%
Ambulatory non-physician services	$422	29%
Outpatient prescribed medicines	$162	57%
Dental services	$295	56%

Source: B. Hahn & D. Lefkowitz, ANNUAL EXPENSES AND SOURCES OF PAYMENT FOR HEALTH CARE SERVICES (Agency for Health Care Policy and Research, Pub. No. 93-0007, 1992) (tables 1 to 7).
[*] As of 1993, this is the most recent year for which such national survey data are available.

hospitals have typically run their enterprises very much like businesses.[16] Normally, they have booked profits, though they do not distribute them to outside owners.

In contrast to Canadians and Europeans, who tightly control the supply side of their health sectors, Americans have generally[17] freely opened theirs to fortune seekers. The American belief is that the GNP transfer that health care providers can extract from the rest of society can easily be controlled through the demand side of the sector—primarily by forcing patients to behave like regular consumers.

The traditional instrument of demand-side cost control in the United States has been cost sharing by patients. As shown in table 3, on average, American patients are not nearly as well insured as is sometimes supposed—not even considering the heyday of the Great Society—though there is a wide dispersion around this average. Some Americans have no health insurance at all, others have very shallow insurance, and some receive from their employers generous coverage that approximates the comprehensive, first-dollar coverage available to Canadians and Europeans. Typical among the latter insured are unionized workers in the northern rust belt.

Even the relatively high degree of cost sharing by American patients, however, has not been able to contain the growth of national health care expenditures.[18] For that reason, additional forms of demand-side controls have been implemented in recent years, namely: (1) ex–post utilization control, (2) prospective and concurrent utilization review by third-party payers (otherwise known as "managed care"), and (3) the so-called preferred provider organizations (PPOs).[19]

A uniquely American form of cost control, aimed more at the supply side of the health care market, is the health maintenance organization (HMO). Basically, the HMO is an insurance contract under which a network of providers is prepaid an annual lump sum capitation per insured in return for the obligation to furnish the insured with all medically necessary care during the contract period. The contract is designed to make providers hold their use of resources in treating patients to the medically necessary minimum. Usually, the HMO contract leads to lower hospitalization rates, other things being equal, and to relatively lower average per capita health care costs.[20] Drawbacks include limiting patient choice among providers and underserving patients.

The Economic Footprints of These Approaches

It is generally agreed, both here and abroad, that the American entrepreneurial approach to health care has begotten one of the most luxurious, dynamic, clinically and organizationally innovative, and technically sophisticated health care systems in the world. At its best, the system has few rivals anywhere, though many health care systems abroad also have facets of genuine excellence. At its worst, however, it has few rivals as well.

The Cost of Health Care

Unfortunately, but perfectly predictably, the open-ended supply side of the American health care system, coupled with a financing system that looks to sick human beings (patients) as major agents of cost control, has led to perennial excess capacity in most parts of the country, and to large and rapidly growing costs. With the exception of New York City and a few states—in which capacity has been tightly controlled through health planning—the average hospital occupancy ratio in the United States is now between 60 and 70%.[21] It is below 50% in some cities.[22] American physicians, for their part, have long deplored a growing physician surplus.[23]

This enormous and excess capacity comes at a stiff price. In 1992, the United States spent close to 14% of its GNP on health care, up from 9.1% in 1980.[24] Current forecasts project a ratio of 18% for the year 2000.[25] By contrast, none of the other industrialized nations currently spends more than 10% of its GNP on health care, and some (the United Kingdom and Japan) spend less than 7%.

It is fair to assert that the high cost of American health care has contributed to a major ethical problem faced by the system. So expensive has American health care become that the nation's middle- and upper-income classes now seem increasingly unwilling to share the blessings of their health care system with their millions of low-income, uninsured fellow citizens. The gentleness and kindness for which Americans had come to be known after World War II has, thus, literally been priced out of the nation's soul. By international standards, American health policy toward the poor—particularly toward poor children—now appears rather callous.

The Uninsured

At this time, some 37 million Americans,[26] over 60% of them full-time employees and their dependents,[27] and more than one-quarter of them children,[28] have no health insurance coverage of any type. Most of these American families have incomes below $20,000 per year.[29] However, for such healthy families, an individually purchased commercial insurance policy with considerable cost sharing can run as high as $4,000 per year.[30] Some insurance companies have ceased to offer the policies even at these prices because they are unprofitable. If such families have chronically ill members, however, a private health insurance policy may not be available to them at all.

Such enormous gaps in health insurance coverage do not occur anywhere else in the industrialized world. As noted above, the other member nations in the Organization for Economic Cooperation and Development (OECD) offer their citizenry universal health insurance coverage for a comprehensive set of health services and supplies, which typically includes dental care and prescription drugs (with the exception of Canada, where these items are covered only for low-income families).[31]

Traditionally, the American health care system has dealt with the uninsured in the following way: for mild to semi-serious illness, care has been effectively rationed on the basis of price and ability to pay. For critically serious illness, however, care has been made available through hospital emergency rooms, which then shift the cost of such charity care (including necessary inpatient care) to paying patients, notably those insured by the business sector.

Unfortunately, in recent years, this source of charity care has begun to disappear. The profit margins of hospitals are squeezed by a combination of excess capacity and downward price pressure by both public and private sector payers. On average, an uninsured, low-income American now receives only about 50 to 70% of the health care that an identical, regularly insured American receives.[32]

Styles of Rationing

The myth that, unlike other nations, America does not ration health care is just that, a myth. Americans do ration health care by price and ability to pay, sometimes in rather disturbing ways.[33] Nations differ from one another not in whether they ration health care—all of them do somehow and in varying degrees—but in their style of rationing and their definition of that very term.

One rationing style is to limit physical capacity and use triage, based on medical judgment and the queue, to determine the allocation of artificially scarce resources among the population.[34] That style of rationing is sometimes referred to as *implicit rationing.* The other style is to ration *explicitly* by price and ability to pay.[35] It is the natural by-product of the so-called "market approach" to health care.

Implicit rationing predominates outside of the United States. In principle, the approach is thought to allocate health care strictly on the basis of medical need, as perceived and ranked by physicians. It is not known whether other variables, such as the patient's social status, ultimately enter the allocation decision as well. For example, one wonders whether a gas station attendant in the United Kingdom has the same degree of access to limited resources as a barrister or university professor who may be able to use social connections to jump the queue.

Many Americans believe that health care is not currently rationed in the United States. That belief seems warranted for well-insured patients who are covered by traditional, open-ended indemnity insurance and living in areas with excess capacity. For many of these patients, there seems to be virtually no limit to the use of real resources in attempts to preserve life or gain certainty in diagnosis.

On the other hand, persons who are less well-insured, uninsured, or

Table 4. Competing Objectives in Health Care: Basic Prototypical
Systems That Span the Set of Actual Systems

Desiderata

Egalitarian Distribution	Freedom from Government Interference in Pricing and in the Practice of Medicine	Budgetary and Cost Control	Prototypical System
Yes	Yes	No	The health care provider's dream world
Yes	No*	Yes	A national health insurance system with fee schedules and other utilization review (e.g., Canada, West Germany)
No*	Yes	Yes	A price-competitive market system

* Trade-off

covered by managed-care plans (including HMOs) do occasionally experience the withholding of health care resources strictly for economic reasons. In fact, in a recent cross-national survey, some 7.5% of the American
respondents (the equivalent of 18 million Americans) claimed that they
had been denied health care for financial reasons.[36] In Canada and the
United Kingdom, fewer than 1% of the survey respondents made that
claim.[37]

Remarkably, the defenders of the American system, who are typically
also vehement detractors of all foreign health systems, generally define
rationing as only the withholding of health care from people who would
have been able and willing to pay for such care with their own money.
It is the nightmare of the well-to-do. Apparently, denial of health care
to needy, uninsured patients who are unable to pay for that care is not
viewed as rationing by these commentators because they have long coun-
tenanced it. How else can one explain these commentators' warnings that
health care in, for example, the Canadian model would lead to rationing
of health care, as if no American were ever denied needed or wanted
health care?

It seems easier to implement the *implicit*, supply-side rationing practiced in most other countries than to use the *explicit* American approach to rationing. For some reason, both physicians and patients appear to accept with greater equanimity the verdict that the necessary capacity is simply not available, rather than the verdict that available, idle capacity will not be made available because some budget has run out.[38] No one likes to see monetary factors enter medical decisions quite so blatantly as explicit rationing requires, yet a nation using the market approach to health care ultimately cannot escape consideration of these factors.

Summary of the Economic Footsteps

There appears to be a trade-off in the organization of health care that simply cannot be avoided. It is a trade-off among three distinct desiderata in health care, namely: (1) the freedom granted health care providers to organize the production of health care and price their products and services as they see fit; (2) the degree of control over total health care expenditures; and (3) the degree of equity attained in the distribution of health care. Table 4 illustrates this trade-off schematically.

The Convergence of Health Care Systems

If one wished to paint with a very broad brush the evolution of health care policy during the past four decades in the industrialized world, one might describe it as a gradual shift from *expenditure-driven financing of health care* to *budget-driven delivery of health care.*

Under expenditure-driven financing, health care providers were allowed to do for patients whatever they saw fit and send the rest of society a bill at prices that seemed "reasonable." Typically, those presented with that bill paid without reservation. If they had reservations, they paid the bill nevertheless because they lacked the countervailing power present in normal markets without third-party payment. Naturally, under this open-ended approach, the supply side of the health sector became a rich economic frontier that attracted both the genius of private entrepreneurship and its relentless search for revenues.

Technological innovation flourished under this approach as the health sector stood an old adage on its head: instead of necessity being the mother of invention, invention became the mother of necessity. Once a technological innovation was at hand, its application was quickly deemed a "medical necessity" as long as it promised any additional benefits at all to the patient.[39] Benefit-cost ratios played no role in this world because the denominator of that ratio—cost—was deemed irrelevant. Indeed, even to consider cost was deemed ethically unacceptable because that consideration might lead to the "rationing" of health care, which was deemed unacceptable on its face.

Under the second approach, budget-driven health care delivery, society establishes some sort of prospective budget for health care and tells providers to do the best they can within that budget. Typically, the establishment of the overall budget has been rather arbitrary in practice, in the sense that the budget is tied to some arbitrary criterion—such as a fixed percentage of the GNP or a fixed annual growth rate.[40] Ideally, this approach should lead policymakers to explore what additional benefits might be gained through incremental budget expansions, and to set the ultimate budget limits accordingly. In any event, however, the application of new medical technologies in this world will typically be subjected to rigorous benefit-cost analysis before payment for such technologies will be made out of the fixed budget. Merely demonstrating promised benefits is no longer sufficient and will not be accepted by those who would stand to lose from applications of novel technology within the given budget constraints.

As noted earlier, most of the industrialized world has already gone a long way toward budget-driven health care delivery, some (England and Sweden, for example) completely. The United States is the odd one out because it is only just beginning to move in that direction. For the most part, both government and private sector payers in the United States are able to figure out what they have spent on health care in any given year with only a lag of a year or so. In fact, the announcement of total national health spending in recent years has lagged behind actual spending by almost two years. The announcement is eagerly anticipated by all concerned, and the actual numbers never cease to surprise.

There seems little doubt, however, that the 1980s represented the last decade of the completely open economic health care frontier in the United States. There is wide agreement in both the public and private sectors that health spending in the United States is out of control and needs to be reigned in by means other than the free market.

Several recent health reform proposals—including the proposal put forth by President Clinton during his campaign, and one by the prestigious American College of Physicians—have called for a global national health care budget.[41] A national board of stakeholders, somewhat akin to

Germany's *Konzertierte Aktion*, determines that budget.[42] At this time, of course, the United States lacks the organizational infrastructure for setting such a budget and apportioning it to the local level. Establishing that infrastructure alone will take over half a decade.

Furthermore, there is already widespread, open hostility toward the very idea of global budgets in the United States, not only among those who define "health care spending" as "health care income." Opponents of global budgeting in the United States offer the strategy of managed competition/managed care as an alternative.[43] Some proponents of that approach market it as the "last hurrah" of the free market, though, in fact, the approach is inherently regulatory in nature.

"Managed competition" is frequently confused with "managed care," but these terms relate to entirely different concepts. "Managed care" refers to the external monitoring and comanaging of an ongoing doctor-patient relationship to ensure that the attending physician prescribes only "appropriate" interventions. The term "appropriate" excludes procedures with no proven medical benefit, but may also eventually exclude beneficial procedures with a low benefit-cost ratio.

"Managed competition," on the other hand, refers to a highly structured and highly regulated framework that forces vertically integrated, income-seeking managed care systems to compete for patients on the basis of prepaid capitation premiums and quality; the latter is to be measured by clinical outcomes and the satisfaction of patients. In other words, the central idea is to put competing managed care systems into transparent, statistical "medico-fishbowls" that can be compared by both patients and those who pay on behalf of patients—for example, government agencies or business firms procuring health insurance coverage for their employees.

At this time, the contrast between the current Canadian/European approach to resource allocation in health care and this newly emerging American approach is stark. Canadians and Europeans still appear to believe that the best way to control overall health spending is to (1) constrain the physical capacity of the health system, (2) control prices, and, for good measure, (3) impose something as close as possible to global monetary budgets on the entire system. Within these constraints, however, they allow doctors and their patients considerable clinical freedom. In this way, the system will tend to maximize the benefits that are wrung out of the constrained set of real and financial resources. In other words, there is considerable trust in the medical establishment's willingness and ability to use the resources made available to it properly, without the need for day-to-day supervision. Direct comanaging of an ongoing patient-doctor relationship in the American model is still rather rare in Canada and Europe.

In contrast, the American proponents of managed competition believe that, by paying for everything that is beneficial, but denying payment for everything else, the nation can avoid setting an arbitrary global budget and will, in the end, devote the "right" percentage of GNP to health care.[44] These proponents have considerable faith in the ability of ordinary consumers to choose wisely among the alternative cost-quality combinations that competing managed-care systems in the health care market offer. On the other hand, they have little faith in the ability or willingness of the individual physician to use scarce resources wisely in the treatment of patients; therefore, they would subject each doctor to constant statistical monitoring and hands-on supervision.[45]

A huge health services research industry has already been busily working on constructing the statistical "fishbowls" that managed competition will require. Whether the American automobile industry will grow in the 1990s is an open question, but the growth of the health services research industry by leaps and bounds seems assured. By the end of the decade, clinical freedom—which older American physicians once knew and loved—will be all but dead. The physicians' daily activities, their successes and failures, will become highly visible blips on sundry computer screens.

Conclusion

And what of the 21st century? How will the health care systems of Canada and Europe compare with the American health care system?

It is my thesis that the current differences between the systems will vanish over time. Most likely, Americans will learn that a managed care/managed competition approach will do many wondrous things, but it will not be able to stop the medical arms race that characterizes the American health system. The proponents of managed competition probably oversell the importance of price in consumers' choices concerning health care. To be sure, price does matter much among low-income households. Nevertheless, it is a safe bet that the competing managed care systems will beckon higher-income households, not chiefly with lower premiums, but with promises of ever-new and abundant medical technology that these elevated economic classes will find irresistible. To deny the well-to-do such novel technology in the American context is very difficult. In the end, those who would be forced to deny it will seek comfortable refuge behind some larger constraint—something like a global national or regional budget. Therefore, the United States health system will eventually envelop the competing medico-fishbowls by a global national budget imposed from the top.

At the same time, however, one must wonder whether countries that could not resist McDonald's hamburgers and Apple computers will be able to resist the magnificent statistical medico-fishbowls now being manufactured all over the United States. There will continue to be top-down budgeting in these countries, but there is apt to be less faith in the ability or willingness of the delivery system to use these budgets and without hands-on supervision. Would it not be nice, and eminently proper, to inquire as to exactly what the little "medico-fish" in the health system actually do with all of the dollars, euros, marks, and pounds poured into these health care systems, particularly when such information is easily retrieved and structured? Should there not be better accountability, by individual doctors and hospitals, for their spending, their clinical outcomes, and the satisfaction they achieve among patients?

Thus, it is my bet that, around the year 2005, the health care systems of Canada and Europe will also be a combination of budgets and statistical medico-fishbowls, and that there will be a brisk commerce of ideas among health services researchers and health care managers across the globe regarding the best ways to construct these medico-fishbowls, behold them, and direct the busy medico-fish within them toward desirable ends. In short, our health systems will converge substantially, bound together by the imperative to constrain the share of GNP allocated to health care, and the awesome capacity of new information technology to extract accountability, even from the hitherto impenetrable health care delivery system.

Notes

1   *See* Uwe E. Reinhardt, *West Germany's Health-Care and Health-Insurance System: Combining Universal Access with Cost Control, in* U.S. Bipartisan Comm'n on Comprehensive Health Care (The Pepper Commission), A Call for Action, 3, 7–9 (Supp. 1990); John K. Iglehart, *Germany's Health Care System*, 324 NEW ENG. J. MED. 503, 503 (1991) (first of two parts).

2   Reinhardt, *supra* note 1, at 7; Iglehart, *supra* note 1, at 503, 504; *see also* Craig R. Whitney, *Paying for Health the German Way*, N.Y. TIMES, Jan. 23, 1993, at 1, 4.

3   *See* Reinhardt, *supra* note 1, at 10–11; Iglehart, *supra* note 1, at 504. The private carriers in

Germany are also subject to considerable federal regulations—among them a government-imposed fee schedule for physicians.

4 Suzanne W. Letsch, *National Health Care Spending in 1991*, HEALTH AFF., Spring 1993, at 94, 101.

5 Jeremy W. Hurst, *Reforming Health Care in Seven European Nations*, HEALTH AFF., Fall 1991, at 9 (reporting results of a study of recent reforms to the health care systems of seven Organization for Economic Cooperation and Development [OECD] countries: Belgium, France, Germany, Ireland, the Netherlands, Spain, and the United Kingdom).

6 *See* Reinhardt, *supra* note 1, at 10. *See also* Iglehart, *supra* note 1, at 507 ("Some 6.3 million Germans—affluent people and many childless couples—purchase comprehensive private insurance."). In Canada, "[p]rivate insurance may cover additional services but duplication of the public coverage is proscribed." Steffie Woolhandler & David U. Himmelstein, *The Deteriorating Administrative Efficiency of the U.S. Health Care System*, 324 NEW ENG. J. MED. 1253, 1253 (1991).

7 *See* Hurst, *supra* note 5, at 12; Eugene Vayda & Raisa B. Deber, *The Canadian Health Care System: A Developmental Overview, in* CANADIAN HEALTH CARE AND THE STATE 125–26 (1992).

8 Hurst, *supra* note 5, at 13–14.

9 *Id.* at 10.

10 General Accounting Office, HEALTH CARE SPENDING CONTROL: THE EXPERIENCE OF FRANCE, GERMANY AND JAPAN 32 (1991).

11 Hurst, *supra* note 5, at 10.

12 *See* Willard G. Manning et al., *Health Insurance and the Demand for Medical Care*, AM. ECON. REV. 251 (1987) (reporting results of the Rand Health Insurance Experiment).

13 *See* Dale A. Rublee, *Medical Technology in Canada, Germany, and the United States*, HEALTH AFF., Fall 1989, at 178, 180 ("American physicians, with a universe of modern technology at their fingertips, are the envy of the world's physicians.").

14 *See* Stuart H. Altman & Marc A. Rodwin, *Halfway Competitive Markets and Ineffective Regulation: The American Health Care System*, 13 J. HEALTH POL., POL'Y & L. 323, 334 (1988). For a discussion of state efforts to control costs, *see* George J. Annas et al., AMERICAN HEALTH LAW 219 (1990).

15 *See* Arnold S. Relman & Uwe E. Reinhardt, *Debating For-Profit Health Care and the Ethics of Physicians*, HEALTH AFF., Summer 1986, at 5, 12. For a general discussion of physician entrepreneurs, see Committee on Implications of For-Profit Enterprise in Health Care, Institute of Medicine, *Physicians and Entrepreneurism in Health Care, in* FOR-PROFIT ENTERPRISE IN HEALTH CARE 151–70 (Bradford H. Gray ed., 1986).

16 Rosemary Stevens, IN SICKNESS AND IN WEALTH: A HISTORY OF THE AMERICAN HOSPITAL IN THE TWENTIETH CENTURY 359–61 (1989).

17 As already noted, some states in the United States control certain segments of their health sector through formal planning—for example, through Certificates-of-Need for hospital beds or hospital-based, high-tech equipment. *See supra* section titled "The Entrepreneurial American Approach." These strictures, however, have generally been of limited effectiveness. Where hospitals have been prohibited from acquiring certain high-tech equipment, for example, physicians have been able to acquire and operate it in close proximity to the hospital without regulatory control.

18 As table 2 suggests, perhaps that particular donkey is just too weak to carry much of a cost-containment load.

19 PPOs are networks of fee-for-service providers that have agreed to grant large, third-party payers price discounts in return for insurance contracts that steer the insured toward these "preferred" providers through specially tailored forms of cost sharing. *See* ANNAS ET AL., *supra* note 14, at 775.

20 *See, e.g.,* Julie Kosterlitz, *Managing Medicaid,* 24 NAT'L L.J. 1111 (1992) (describing how HMOs have lower per capita health care costs than does Medicaid in Ohio).

21 Edmund F. Haislmaier, *Why Global Budgets and Price Controls Will Not Curb Health Costs,* HERITAGE FOUND. REP., Mar. 8, 1993, *available in* LEXIS, Nexis Library, Omni File.

22 *See* George D. Pillari, *Those Pliable Occupancy Rates,* MOD. HEALTHCARE, May 20, 1991, at 26, 27 (listing 1990's median occupancy rate for 5600 U.S. hospitals at 48.85%).

23 Kevin Grumbach & Philip Lee, *How Many Physicians Can We Afford,* 265 JAMA 2369, 2369 (1991).

24 *See* Erik Eckholm, *Those Who Pay Health Costs Think About Drawing Lines,* N.Y. TIMES, Mar. 28, 1993, § 4, at 1.

25 Congressional Budget Office, PROJECTION OF NATIONAL HEALTH EXPENDITURES 1 (1992); *see also* Dana Priest, *Health Care Price Caps Considered,* WASH. POST, Feb. 14, 1993, at A1.

26 Glenn Kessler, *Bitter Medicine: Reform Is Coming—and This Could Be Painful,* NEWSDAY, Apr. 11, 1993, at 11.

27 BNA, *Number of Uninsured Persons Increased to 36.6 Million in 1991,* DAILY LABOR REP., Jan. 12, 1993, *available in* LEXIS, Nexis Library, Omni file (reporting results of the Employee Benefit Research Institute Study).

28 M. Susan Marquis & Stephen H. Long, *Uninsured Children and National Health Reform,* 268 JAMA 3473, 3473 (1992).

29 BNA, *supra* note 27; *see also* David U. Himmelstein et al., *The Vanishing Health Care Safety Net: New Data on Uninsured Americans,* 22 INT'L J. HEALTH SVCS. 381, 387 (1992).

30 *See, e.g.,* Susan Dentzer, *Health Care Gridlock,* U.S. NEWS & WORLD REP., Jan. 20, 1992, at 22; Lynn Wagner, *Health Economist Trashes Reform Plans of Both Bush and Clinton,* MOD. HEALTHCARE, Oct. 12, 1992, at 10.

31 *See* Raisa B. Deber, *Canadian Medicare: Can It Work in the United States? Will It Survive in Canada?,* 19 AM. J. L. & MED. 75, 79 (1993). For a discussion about Canada's funding drugs for low-income families, see *supra* Section II.A.

32 *See* U.S. Bipartisan Comm'n on Comprehensive Health Care (The Pepper Commission), A CALL FOR ACTION 34–35 (1990).

33 For example, "[o]ne obstetrician . . . said she doesn't inform pregnant Medicaid patients that they are entitled to a pain killing epidural while in labor [because] Medicaid reimbursements to anesthesiologists are so low, they balk at taking her patients." Kinsey Wilson, *Nobody Likes the R-Word: Rationing of Care Is Unpopular, but It's Happening Just the Same,* NEWSDAY, Apr. 22, 1993, at 23.

34 *See, e.g.,* Richard E. Brown, *From Advocacy to Allocation: The Evolving American Health Care System,* 316 NEW ENG. J. MED. 169 (1987).

35 *See, e.g.,* David Kirkpatrick, *Practicing Medicine above and below the 49th Parallel; One Physician's Experience: The Fiction, the Facts,* 151 ARCH. INTERN. MED. 2150, 2152 (1991).

36 Robert J. Blendon, *Views on Health Care: Public Opinion in Three Nations*, HEALTH AFF., Spring 1989, at 151, 156.

37 *Id.*

38 In this regard, see the fascinating analysis of this facet of British health care in Henry J. Aaron & William B. Schwartz, THE PAINFUL PRESCRIPTION: RATIONING HOSPITAL CARE (1984).

39 For a discussion of the "career" of a medical technology innovation, see John B. McKinlay, *From "Promising Report" to "Standard Procedure": Seven Stages in the Career of a Medical Innovation*, 59 MILBANK MEM. FUND Q. 374 (1981).

40 For example, Germany's health care spending limit is tied to the growth of workers' salaries and wages. *See* John K. Iglehart, *Germany's Health Care System*, 324 NEW ENG. J. MED. 1750, 1751 (1991) (second of two parts).

41 For a description of this aspect of the Clinton proposal, see Uwe E. Reinhardt, *Commentary: Politics and the Health Care System*, 327 NEW ENG. J. MED. 809, 811 (1992). The American College of Physicians's proposal was first outlined in American College of Physicians, *Universal Insurance for American Health Care*, 117 ANN. INTERN. MED. 511 (1992).

42 *Konzertierte Aktion*, or the Concerted Action Conference, is a group that recommends the annual aggregate increases in providers' fees and suppliers' prices. Iglehart, *supra* note 40, at 1752.

43 *See, e.g.*, Alain C. Enthoven, *Commentary: Measuring the Candidates on Health Care*, 327 NEW ENG. J. MED. 807 (1992). For a discussion of one of Enthoven's proposals, see John B. Judis, *Whose Managed Competition?*, NEW REPUBLIC, Mar. 29, 1993, at 22–23. For a critical review of the concept of managed competition, see Uwe E. Reinhardt, *Comment on the Jackson Hole Initiatives for a Twenty-First Century American Health Care System*, HEALTH ECON., Apr. 1993, at 7.

44 *See* Alain C. Enthoven, *The History and Principles of Managed Competition*, HEALTH AFF., Supp. 1993, at 24, 29.

45 Alan L. Hillman et al., *Safeguarding Quality in Managed Competition*, HEALTH AFF., Supp. 1993, at 110 (discussing strategies for implementing a system of quality assurance under managed competition).

Health Care in Four Nations

Thomas Bodenheimer and Kevin Grumbach

The financing and organization of medical care throughout the developed world spans a broad spectrum (Roemer, 1993). In most countries, the preponderance of medical care is financed or delivered (or both) in the public sector; in others, like the United States, most people both pay for and receive their care through private institutions.

In this essay, we describe the health care systems of four nations: Germany, Canada, the United Kingdom, and Japan. Each of these nations resides at a different point on the international health care continuum. Examining their diverse systems may aid us in our search for a suitable health care system for the United States.

Recall the four varieties of health care financing: out-of-pocket payments, individual private insurance, employment-based private insurance, and government financing. Germany, Canada, the United Kingdom, and Japan use the first two modes of payment only to a minimal degree. Germany finances medical care through government-mandated, employment-based private insurance, though German private insurance is a world apart from that found in the United States. Canada and the United Kingdom use essentially government-financed systems. Japan's financing falls between the German method of private financing and the government model of Canada and the United Kingdom. Regarding the delivery of medical care, the German, Japanese, and Canadian systems are predominantly private, while the United Kingdom's is largely public.

Although these four nations demonstrate great differences in their manner of financing and organizing medical care, in one respect they are

Thomas Bodenheimer and Kevin Grumbach, "Health Care in Four Nations," from *Understanding Health Policy*, 160–175. © 2002 by McGraw-Hill/Appleton and Lange. Reprinted by permission of the publisher.

identical: they all provide universal health care coverage, thereby guaranteeing to their populations access to medical services.

Germany

Health Insurance

Hans Deutsch is a bank teller living in Germany (formerly West Germany). He and his family receive health insurance through a sickness fund that insures other employees and their families at his bank and at other workplaces in his city. When Hans went to work at the bank, he was required by law to join the sickness fund selected by his employer.

The bank contributes 7% of Hans's salary to the sickness fund, and an additional 7% is withheld from Hans's paycheck and sent to the fund. Hans's sickness fund collects the same 14% employer–employee contribution for all its members. Some bank employees were grumbling two years ago because the sickness fund raised the rate from 12% to 14%, but Hans feels relatively lucky. He has friends in other sickness funds whose contribution rate is 16%, half from employer and half from employee.

Germany was the first nation to enact compulsory health insurance legislation. Its pioneering law of 1883 required certain employers and employees to make payments to existing voluntary sickness funds, which would pay for the covered employees' medical care. Initially, only industrial wage earners with incomes less than $500 per year were included; the eligible population was extended in later years.

About 90% of Germans now receive their health insurance through the mandatory sickness funds (figure 1). Most people belong to the same fund throughout their lives, although switching does take place. Several categories of sickness funds exist. Forty percent of people (mostly blue-collar workers and their families) belong to funds organized by geographic area; 27% (for the most part the families of white-collar workers) are in nationally based "substitute" funds; 12% are employees or dependents of employees who work in 700 companies that have their own sickness funds; and another 12% are in funds covering all workers in a particular craft.

The sickness funds are nonprofit, closely regulated entities that lie

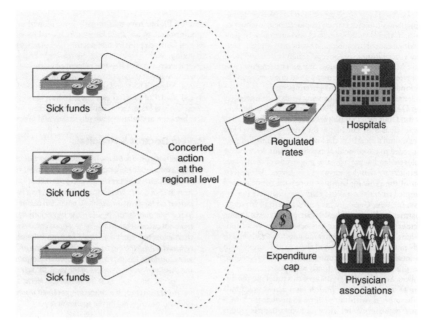

Sick funds

Sick funds

Sick funds

Concerted
action
at the
regional level

Regulated
rates

Hospitals

Expenditure
cap

Physician
associations

Figure 1. The German National Health Insurance System

somewhere between the private and public sectors. The funds collect money from their members and their members' employers and pay for the care of their members. About 500 sickness funds exist in Germany (Brown and Amelung, 1999). The funds are not allowed to exclude people due to illness, or to raise contribution rates according to age or medical condition, i.e., they may not use experience rating. The funds are required to cover a broad range of benefits, including hospital and physician services, prescription drugs, and dental, preventive, and maternity care. Copayments are modest (Iglehart, 1991).

Hans's father, Peter Deutsch, is retired from his job as a machinist in a steel plant. When he worked, his family received health insurance through a sickness fund set up for employees of the steel company. The fund was run by a board, half of whose members represented employees and the other half the employer. On retirement, Peter's family continued its coverage through the same sickness fund, with no change in benefits. The sickness fund continues to pay about 60% of his family's health care costs (subsidized by the contributions of active workers and the employer), with 40% paid from Peter's retirement pension fund.

Hans has a cousin, Georg, who formerly worked for a gas station in Hans's city but is now unemployed. Georg remained in his sickness fund after losing his job. His contribution to the fund is paid by the government. Hans's best friend at the bank was diagnosed with lymphoma and became permanently disabled and unable to work. He remained in the sickness fund, with his contribution paid by the government.

Upon retiring from or losing a job, people and their families retain membership in their sickness funds. Health insurance in Germany, as in the United States, is employment based; but German health insurance, unlike in the United States, must continue to cover its members whether or not they change jobs or stop working for any reason.

Hans's Uncle Karl is an assistant vice president at the bank. Because he earns over $40,000 per year, he is not required to join a sickness fund, but can opt to purchase private health insurance. If he chooses private insurance, he will not be able to enter a sickness fund in the future. Most higher-paid employees choose a sickness fund; they are not required to join the fund selected by the employer for lower paid workers, but can join one of 15 national "substitute" funds.

Eight percent of Germans, all with incomes over $40,000, choose private insurance. Private insurers pay substantially higher fees to physicians than do the sickness funds, often allowing their policyholders to receive preferential treatment when seeing a physician (Iglehart, 1991). In summary, in Germany, 90% of the populace belong to the mandatory sickness fund system, 8% opt for private insurance, 2% receive medical services as members of the armed forces or police, and less than 0.2% (all of whom are wealthy) have no coverage (Saltman, 1988; Files and Murray, 1995).

Germany finances health care through a merged social insurance and public assistance structure, such that no distinctions are made between employed people who contribute to their health insurance, and unemployed people, whose contribution is made by the government. Germany's social insurance concept is slightly different from that of Medicare in the United States: The employer and employee payments in Germany go to quasi-public sickness funds rather than to the government.

Germany's method of financing tends to be regressive. Hans Deutsch contributes 7% of his paycheck to his sickness fund, but other employees contribute as little as 4% or as much as 8%. The higher the average wage level of a sickness fund's members, the lower the percentage of payroll needed to cover medical expenses. Thus, lower-wage employees tend to pay a greater proportion of their wages for health care than higher-wage employees. An appreciation of the growing inequity in payroll contributions prompted recent reforms in health care financing in Germany. In 1994, Germany instituted a method to reduce disparities in the rate of health care payroll taxes among different sick funds. Under this new system, sick funds that have enrollees with higher incomes and lower health needs must refund a portion of their payroll revenues to a national pool. The government then distributes money from this risk pool to sick funds with poorer and sicker enrollees. Since implementation of this program, the differential in payroll contribution rates across sick funds has diminished, with rates falling somewhat for lower-income populations and rising for higher-income groups (Files and Murray, 1995).

Medical Care

> Hans Deutsch develops chest pain while walking, and it worries him. He does not have a physician, and a friend recommends a general practitioner (GP), Dr. Helmut Arzt. Because Hans is free to see any ambulatory care physician he chooses, he indeed visits Dr. Arzt, who diagnoses angina pectoris—coronary artery disease. Dr. Arzt prescribes some medications and a low-fat diet, but the pain persists. One morning, Hans awakens with severe, suffocating chest pain. He calls Dr. Arzt, who orders an ambulance to take Hans to a nearby hospital. Hans is admitted for a heart attack, and is cared for by Dr. Edgar Hertz, a cardiologist. Dr. Arzt does not visit Hans in the hospital. Upon discharge, Dr. Hertz sends a report to Dr. Arzt, who then resumes Hans's medical care. Hans never receives a bill.

German medicine maintains a strict separation of ambulatory care physicians and hospital-based physicians. Most ambulatory care physicians are prohibited from treating patients in hospitals, and most hospital-based physicians do not have private offices for treating outpatients. People often have their own primary care physician (PCP), but have traditionally been allowed to make appointments to see ambulatory care specialists without referral from the primary care doctor. This practice is now changing, with specialty visits increasingly requiring a referral from a PCP. Fifty-five percent of Germany's physicians are generalists, compared with only 35% in the United States. The German system tends to use the dispersed model of medical care organization characteristic of the United States, with little coordination between ambulatory care physicians and hospitals.

Paying Doctors and Hospitals

> Dr. Arzt was used to billing his regional association of physicians and receiving a fee for each patient visit and for each procedure done during the visit. In 1986, he was shocked to find that spending caps had been placed on the total ambulatory physician budget. If in the first quarter of the year, the physicians in his regional association billed for more patient services than expected, each fee would be proportionately reduced during the next quarter. If the volume of services continued to increase, fees would drop again in the third and fourth quarters of the year. Dr. Arzt discussed the situation with his friend, Dr. Hertz, but Dr. Hertz, as a hospital physician, received a salary and was not affected by the spending cap.

Ambulatory care physicians are required to join their regional physicians' association. Rather than paying physicians directly, sickness funds pay a global sum each year to the physicians' association in their region, which in turn pays physicians on the basis of a detailed fee schedule. Since 1986, physicians' associations, in an attempt to stay within their global budgets, have reduced fees on a quarterly basis if the volume of services delivered by their physicians was too high. Sickness funds pay hospitals on a basis similar to the diagnosis-related groups used in the U.S. Medicare program. Included within this payment is the salary of hospital-based physicians.

Cost Control

Between 1965 and 1975, West German health care costs flew out of control, rising from 5.1% to 7.8% of the gross domestic product. As a remedy, the government intervened by passing the 1977 Cost Containment Act. This law imposed a number of fiscal restrictions and created a body called Concerted Action, made up of representatives of the nation's health providers, sickness funds, employers, unions, and different levels of government. Concerted Action is convened twice each year, and every spring it sets guidelines for physician fees, hospital rates, and the prices of pharmaceuticals and other supplies. Based on these guidelines, negotiations are conducted at state, regional, and local levels between the sickness funds in a region, the regional physicians' association, and the hospitals to set physician fees and hospital rates that reflect Concerted Action guidelines. Since 1986, not only have physician fees been controlled, but, as described in the above vignette about Dr. Arzt, the total amount of money flowing to physicians has been capped. As a result of these efforts, Germany's health expenditures as a percentage of the gross domestic product actually fell between 1985 and 1991, from 8.7% to 8.5% (Schieber et al., 1993).

Germany's cost control troubles, however, are not over. In 1991, health care costs had a new upward surge, paving the way for a 1993 cost control law restricting the growth of sickness fund budgets. Faced with persistent cost increases, Germany recently attempted to inject more competition into its insurance system by allowing individuals greater flexibility in choosing a sickness fund, rather than being limited to the sickness fund associated with their employment or municipality. The expectation was that individuals would seek out lower cost sick funds and that this "consumer choice" dynamic would motivate all sick funds to become more price competitive. However, Germans have shown considerable allegiance to their traditional sick funds, and few have switched plans under the new laws. German health care values of social solidarity and fairness have tended to dampen aggressive price competition and shopping for health plans (Brown and Amelung, 1999). In 1998 health care costs were 10.6% of GDP, second only to the United States.

Canada

Health Insurance

The Maple family owns a small grocery store in Outer Snowshoe, a tiny Canadian town. Grandfather Maple has a heart condition for which he sees Dr. Rebecca North, his family physician, regularly. The rest of the family is healthy and goes to Dr. North for minor problems and preventive care, including children's immunizations. Neither as employers nor as health consumers do the Maples worry about health insurance. They receive a plastic card from their provincial government and show the card when they visit Dr. North.

The Maples do worry about taxes. The federal personal income tax, the 1991 goods and services tax, and the various provincial taxes take almost 40% of the family's income. But the Maples would never let anyone take away their health insurance system.

In 1947, the province of Saskatchewan initiated the first publicly financed universal hospital insurance program in North America. Other provinces followed suit, and in 1957, the Canadian government passed the Hospital Insurance Act, which was fully implemented by 1961. Hospital, but not physician, services were covered. In 1963, Saskatchewan again took the lead and enacted a medical insurance plan for physician services. The Canadian federal government passed universal medical insurance in 1966; the program was fully operational by 1971 (Taylor, 1990).

Canada has a tax-financed, public, single-payer health care system. In each Canadian province, the single payer is the provincial government (figure 2). During the 1970s, federal taxes financed 50% of health services, but since the 1980s, the provinces have had to pay medical costs increasing above the gross national product's growth rate. By 1996, federal tax transfers supported only 22% of provincial health plan costs (Naylor, 1999). Provincial taxes vary in type from province to province and include income taxes, payroll taxes, and sales taxes. Two provinces, British Columbia and Alberta, charge a compulsory health care premium to finance a small portion of their health budgets.

Canada, unlike Germany, has severed the link between employment and health insurance. Wealthy or poor, employed or jobless, retired or under age 18, every Canadian receives the same health insurance, financed in the same way. No Canadian would even imagine that leaving, changing, retiring from, or losing a job has anything to do with health insurance. In Canada, no distinction is made between the two public financing mechanisms of social insurance (in which only those who contribute receive benefits) and public assistance (in which people receive benefits based on need rather than on having contributed). Everyone contributes through the tax structure and everyone receives benefits.

The benefits provided by Canadian provinces are broad, including unlimited hospital, physician, and ancillary services. Provincial plans also pay for outpatient drugs, although most provinces limit eligibility for this benefit to elderly and low-income patients. Long-term care benefits also vary from province to province.

The Canadian health care system is unique in its prohibition of private

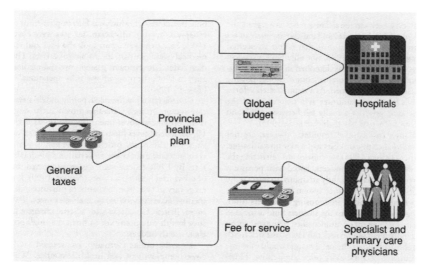

Figure 2. The Canadian National Health Insurance System

health insurance for coverage of services included in the provincial health plans. Hospitals and physicians that receive payments from the provincial health plans are not allowed to bill private insurers for such services, thereby avoiding the preferential treatment of privately insured patients that occurs in many health care systems. A small number of upper-income Canadians purchase health insurance policies for the few gaps in provincial health plan coverage or for such amenities as private hospital rooms.

Medical Care

Grandfather Maple wakes up one morning with a feeling of palpitations in his chest. He calls Dr. North, who tells him to come right over. An electrocardiogram reveals rapid atrial fibrillation, an abnormal heart rhythm. Because Mr. Maple is tolerating the rapid rhythm, Dr. North treats him with digoxin in the office, tells him to return the next day, and writes out a referral slip to see Dr. Jonathan Hartwell, the cardiologist in a nearby small city.

Dr. Hartwell arranges a stress echocardiogram at the local hospital to evaluate Mr. Maple's arrhythmia, finds severe coronary ischemia, and explains to Mr. Maple that his coronary arteries are narrowed. He recommends a coronary angiogram and possible coronary artery bypass surgery. Because Mr. Maple's condition is not urgent, Dr. Hartwell arranges for his patient to be placed on the waiting list at the University Hospital in the provincial capital 50 miles away. One month later, Mr. Maple awakens at 2 a.m. in a cold sweat, gasping for breath. His daughter calls Dr. North, who urgently sends for an ambulance to transport Mr. Maple to the University Hospital. There, Mr. Maple is admitted to the coronary care unit, his condition is stabilized, and he undergoes emergency coronary artery bypass surgery the next day. Ten days later, Mr. Maple returns home, complaining of pain in his incision but otherwise feeling well.

Fifty-five percent of Canadian physicians are GPs or family practitioners who act as gatekeepers to the medical care delivery system. Canadians have free choice of physician. As a rule, Canadians see their GP for routine medical problems and visit specialists only through referral by the GP. Specialists are allowed to see patients without referrals, but only receive the higher specialist fee if they include the referral slip in their billing; for that reason, most specialists will not see patients without a referral. Because 55% of Canadian physicians are GPs or family practitioners (contrasted with the United States, where only 35% of physicians are generalists), primary care services are in ample supply, except in remote rural areas. Elderly Canadians receive 17% more physician services than the elderly in the United States (Welch et al., 1996). Unlike the European model of separation between ambulatory and hospital physicians, Canadian family physicians are allowed to care for their patients in hospitals, although they tend to perform less inpatient work than U.S. family physicians.

Because of the close scientific interchange between Canada and the United States, the practice of Canadian medicine is similar to that in the United States; the differences lie in the financing system and the far greater use of PCPs as gatekeepers. The treatment of Mr. Maple's heart condition is not significantly different from what would occur in the United States, with two exceptions:

(1) High-technology procedures such as cardiac surgery and MRI scans are regionalized in a limited number of facilities and performed less frequently than in the United States (Grumbach et al., 1995; Anderson et al., 1993; Katz et al., 1996a); and

(2) There are waiting lists for some specialized elective procedures. The average patient scheduled for a knee-replacement operation in Ontario in

the late 1980s waited eight weeks, compared with a three-week wait for the average patient in the United States (Coyte et al., 1994). On the other hand, patients diagnosed with leukemia in Canada did not wait longer to receive bone marrow transplantation than patients in the United States with the same condition (Silberman et al., 1994).

Although Canadians may in some instances wait longer for operations than do insured people in the United States, Canada's universal insurance program has created a fairer system for distributing health services. Studies of the United States and Canada have compared how receipt of a variety of services, ranging from cardiac surgery to mental health care, may vary according to income in the two nations. These studies indicate that in the United States, people with higher incomes tend to use more services, but no similar differential according to income exists in Canada for most services studied. In some cases, lower-income groups in Canada are the *most* likely to receive health services such as cardiac surgery, a pattern that corresponds to the higher burden of disease among lower-income groups (Anderson et al., 1993; Katz et al., 1996b; Katz et al., 1997).

Paying Doctors and Hospitals

> For Dr. Rebecca North, collecting fees is a simple matter. Each week she sends a computer disk to the provincial government, listing the patients she saw and the services she provided. Within a month, she is paid in full, according to a fee schedule. Dr. North wishes the fees were higher, but loves the simplicity of the billing process. Her staff spends 2 hours per week on billing, compared with the 30 hours of staff time her friend Dr. South in Michigan needs for billing purposes.
>
> Dr. North is less happy about the global budget approach used to pay hospitals. She often begs the hospital administrator to hire more physical therapists, to speed up the reporting of laboratory results, and to institute a program of diabetic teaching. The administrator responds that he receives a fixed payment from the provincial government each year, and there is no extra money.

Physicians in Canada—GPs and specialists—are paid on a fee-for-service basis, with fee levels negotiated between provincial governments and provincial medical associations (figure 2). Previously, physicians were allowed to bill patients in addition to billing the government; this practice was prohibited in 1984 (Lomas et al., 1989). Canadian hospitals, most of which are private nonprofit institutions, negotiate a global budget with the provincial government each year. Hospitals have no need to prepare the itemized patient bills that are so administratively costly in the United States. Hospitals must receive approval from their provincial health plan for new capital projects such as the purchase of expensive new technology or the construction of new facilities. Canada also regulates pharmaceutical prices and provincial plans maintain formularies of drugs approved for coverage.

Cost Control

The Canadian system has attracted the interest of many people in the United States because, in contrast to the United States, the Canadians have found a way to deliver comprehensive care to their entire population at far less cost. In 1970, the year before Canada's single-payer system was fully in place, Canada and the United States spent approximately the same proportion of their gross domestic products on health care—7.2% and 7.4% respectively. By 1991, Canada's health expenditures had risen to 10% of the gross domestic product, compared with 13.2% for the United States. Since 1991, Canada's health care costs have actually declined, compared with continued cost increases in the United States. In 1998, Canada spent 9.5% of its gross domestic product on health care; the United States spent 13.6%. The 1998 per capita cost of health care in the United States was 80% higher than the per capita cost in Canada (Anderson and Hussey, 2001).

Notably, the differences in cost between the United States and Canada are not a result of Canadians receiving fewer services overall. In fact, Canadians on the average spend more days in the hospital and see physicians more often than people in the United States. Lower costs in Canada are primarily accounted for by three items: (1) administrative costs, which are 300% greater per capita in the United States; (2) cost per patient day in hospitals, which reflects a greater intensity of service in the United States; and (3) physician fees and pharmaceutical prices, which are much higher in the United States (Evans et al., 1989; Fuchs and Hahn, 1990; Woolhandler and Himmelstein, 1991; Menon, 2001).

Viewed from across its southern border, Canada appears to be doing well in containing health care costs, but within Canada, costs are seen as a serious problem. After all, aside from the United States, Canada has one of the most expensive health care systems in the world. Health expenditures account for about one-third of provincial budgets. Rising taxes and governmental budget deficits are attributable in part to health care inflation. Some Canadian analysts feel that the fee-for-service method of paying physicians is a major impetus to health cost inflation (Evans, 1990; Rachlis and Kushner, 1989). As a remedy for its inflation problem, all provinces have put into effect caps on physician payments similar to those used in Germany (Barer et al., 1996).

The United Kingdom

Health Insurance

> Roderick Pound owns a small bicycle repair shop in the north of England; he lives with his wife and two children. His sister Jennifer is a lawyer in Scotland. Roderick's younger brother is a student at Oxford, and their widowed mother, a retired saleswoman, lives in London. Their cousin Anne is totally and permanently disabled from a tragic automobile accident. A distant relative, who became a U.S. citizen 15 years before, recently arrived to help care for Anne.
>
> Simply by virtue of existing on the soil of the United Kingdom—whether employed, retired, disabled, or a foreign visitor—each of the Pound family members is entitled to receive tax-supported medical care through the National Health Service (NHS).

In 1911, Great Britain established a system of health insurance similar to that of Germany. About half the population was covered, and the insurance arrangements were highly complex, with contributions flowing to "friendly societies," trade union and employer funds, commercial insurers, and county insurance committees. In 1942, the world's most renowned treatise on social insurance was published by Sir William Beveridge. The Beveridge Report proposed that Britain's diverse and complex social insurance and public assistance programs, including retirement, disability and unemployment benefits, welfare payments, and medical care, be financed and administered in a simple and uniform system. One part of Beveridge's vision was the creation of a national health service for the entire population. In 1948, the NHS began (Sidel and Sidel, 1983).

Eighty-two percent of NHS funding comes from taxes, 13% from employer-employee contributions similar to social security payments in the United States, and 4% from user charges (Maynard and Bloor, 1996). As

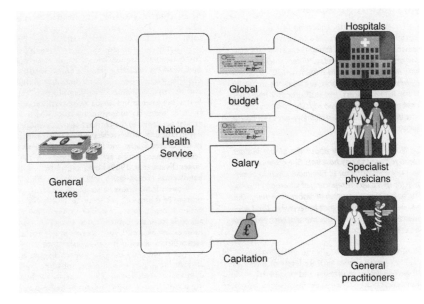

Figure 3. The British National Health Service: Traditional Model

in Canada, the United Kingdom completely separates health insurance from employment, and no distinction exists between social insurance and public assistance financing. Unlike Canada, the United Kingdom allows private insurance companies to sell health insurance for services also covered by the NHS. A number of affluent people purchase private insurance in order to receive preferential treatment, "hopping over" the queues for services present in parts of the NHS (Lister, 1988). Some employers offer such supplemental insurance as a perk. Naturally, the 11% of the population with private insurance are also paying taxes to support the NHS (figure 3).

Medical Care

Dr. Timothy Broadman is an English GP, whose list of patients numbers 1750. Included on his list is Roderick Pound and his family. One day, Roderick's son broke his leg playing soccer. He was brought to the NHS district hospital by ambulance and treated by Dr. Pettibone, the hospital orthopedist, without ever seeing Dr. Broadman.

Roderick's mother has severe degenerative arthritis of the hip, which Dr. Broadman cares for. A year ago, Dr. Broadman sent her to Dr. Pettibone to be evaluated for a hip replacement. Because this was not an emergency, Mrs. Pound required a referral from Dr. Broadman to see Dr. Pettibone. The orthopedist examined and X-rayed her hip and agreed that she needed a hip replacement, but not on an urgent basis. Mrs. Pound has been on the waiting list for her surgery for over six months. Mrs. Pound has a wealthy friend with private health insurance who got her hip replacement within three weeks from Dr. Pettibone, who has a private practice in addition to his employment with the NHS.

Prior to the NHS, most primary medical care was delivered through GPs. The NHS maintained this tradition and formalized a gatekeeper system by which specialty and hospital services (except in emergencies) are available only by referral from a GP. Every person in the United Kingdom who wants to use the NHS must be enrolled on the list of a GP. There is free choice of GP (unless the GP's list of patients is full), and people can (but rarely do) switch from one GP's list to another.

Whereas the creation of the NHS in 1948 left primary care essentially unchanged, it revolutionized Britain's hospital sector. As in the United States, hospitals had mainly been private nonprofit institutions or were run by local government; most of these hospitals were nationalized and arranged into administrative regions. Because the NHS unified the United Kingdom's hospitals under the national government, it was possible to institute a true regionalized plan.

Patient flow in a regionalized system tends to go from GP (primary care for common illnesses) to local hospital (secondary care for more serious illnesses) to regional or national teaching hospital (tertiary care for complex illnesses). Traditionally, most specialists have had their offices in hospitals. As in Germany, GPs do not provide care in hospitals. GPs have a tradition of working closely with social service agencies in the community, and home care is highly developed in the United Kingdom (Sidel and Sidel, 1983).

Paying Doctors and Hospitals

Dr. Timothy Broadman does not think much about money when he goes to his surgery (office) each morning. He receives a payment from the NHS to cover part of the cost of running his office, and every month he receives a capitation payment for each of the 1,750 patients on his list. Because he cannot influence the number of people on his list, there isn't much he can do to change his income. Recently, 10% of his income has been coming from extra fees he receives when he gives vaccinations to the kids and does Pap smears, family planning, and other preventive care. He also gets extra payment for making home visits after hours. There is no particular reason for money to be on Dr. Broadman's mind when he cares for his patients.

Since early in the 20th century, the major method of payment for British GPs has been capitation. This mode of payment did not change when the NHS took over in 1948. The NHS did add some fee-for-service payments as an encouragement to provide certain preventive services and home visits during nights and weekends. Consultants (specialists) are salaried employees of the NHS, though some consultants are allowed to see privately insured patients on the side, whom they bill fee-for-service.

Cost Control

Health expenditures in the United Kingdom accounted for 5.9% of the gross domestic product in 1985 and 6.7% in 1998. In 1998, United Kingdom per capita health spending was only 35% of the U.S. figure (Anderson and Hussey, 2001).

Two major factors allow the United Kingdom to keep its health care costs low: the power of the governmental single payer to limit budgets and the mode of reimbursement of physicians. While Canada also has a single payer of health services, it pays most physicians fee-for-service and only recently has moved toward physician expenditure caps (like Germany) in an attempt to control the inflationary tendencies of fee-for-service reimbursement. The United Kingdom, in contrast, relies chiefly on capitation and salary to pay physicians; payment can more easily be controlled by limiting increases in capitation payments and salaries. Moreover, because consultants (specialists) in the United Kingdom are NHS employees, the NHS can and does tightly restrict the number of consultant slots, including those for surgeons. As a result, queues have developed for nonemergency consultant visits, and the rates of some forms of the surgery such as gallbladder operations are half those in the United States and Canada (Hiatt, 1987). Overall, the United Kingdom controls costs by controlling the supply of personnel and facilities and the budget for medical resources.

Critics both within and outside the United Kingdom suggest that health care costs are controlled too tightly (Lister, 1988; Aaron and Schwartz, 1984). In the 1980s, the Thatcher government strictly limited the rate of growth of the NHS budget. In the late 1980s, underpaid nurses were leaving employment at the rate of 30,000 per year. Even with hospital beds, operating theaters, and surgeons available, the shortage of skilled nurses caused increases in queues. For the first time, the overwhelming public support for the NHS was beginning to erode (Lister, 1988).

In light of the low level of health expenditures, the United Kingdom is often viewed as a nation that rations certain kinds of health care. In fact, primary and preventive care are not rationed, and average waiting times to see a GP are probably shorter than delays for similar appointments in many parts of the United States. Even some high-technology services (e.g., radiation therapy for cancer and bone marrow transplantation) are performed at the same rates as in the United States. But waiting times to see consultants for nonurgent problems, elective hospital admissions, and such elective surgeries as hip replacement and cataract removal may be substantial (though 90% of elective waits are under three months) (Potter and Porter, 1989). Renal dialysis is performed far less often in the United Kingdom than in the United States, especially for people over 60 years of age, a practice that has been criticized by U.S. observers (Aaron and Schwartz, 1984). Overall, a striking characteristic of British medicine is its economy. British physicians simply do less of nearly everything—perform fewer surgeries, prescribe fewer medications, and order fewer X-rays. They are more skeptical of new technologies than U.S. physicians (Payer, 1988).

The single-payer form of health care system, as the United Kingdom exemplifies, is capable of keeping health expenditures down. However, not all single-payer health care systems have low per capita costs: Canada's per capita expenditures are relatively high. In part, the United Kingdom dedicates less to health care because of its poor economy. As a general rule, nations such as the United Kingdom, with a low gross domestic product per capita, spend a smaller portion of that gross domestic product on health care.

Recent Reforms of the NHS

Nagging problems such as long surgical waiting lists have been a political thorn in the side for several British prime ministers, with campaign pledges of a new and improved NHS featuring prominently in recent national elections. In 1990, Conservative prime minister Margaret Thatcher launched a major policy initiative to introduce more competition into the NHS in an attempt to stimulate greater efficiency and patient responsiveness. Soon after his election in 1997, Labour prime minister Tony Blair issued his own briefing paper for NHS reform, entitled "The New NHS: Modern, Dependable," which softened some of the competitive edges of the Thatcher policies while continuing to reorganize aspects of the NHS and increasing NHS funding. Although none of these reforms, whether from conservative or liberal administrations, has fundamentally altered the basic tenets of the NHS as a publicly financed, universal health care system, they have restructured the organization of the NHS.

One outcome of these many reforms has been to give hospitals greater budgetary and managerial autonomy, with less direct control from regional NHS administrative agencies. In principle, hospitals must now be more accountable for the quality and timeliness of the services they provide, with NHS agencies having more flexibility to shift funding to different hospitals on the basis of hospital performance.

General practice has undergone continual revision over the past decade. Under the Thatcher pro-competition policies, GP practices could opt for more of a U.S. style of capitation contract, known as "GP fund holding." Under fund holding, GP practices were given an expanded capitation budget to allow GPs to purchase specialty and ancillary services for their patients, in addition to funding primary care GP services. GP practices were permitted to retain any surpluses in their fund-holding budgets, although they were required to reinvest this surplus in improvements in their practice rather than pocketing the money as additional personal income, as occurs in similar types of capitation arrangements in the U.S. Nonetheless, GP fund holding generated many of the same objections about physicians' financial conflict of interest and incentives to avoid high-cost patients that have been leveled at high-risk capitation contracts in the United States.

The Blair reforms eliminated GP fund holding while introducing a new strategy to increase GP involvement in budgetary planning and promote greater GP accountability for quality of care. Since 1999, all GPs in England within a designated geographic area have been required to become members of their local primary care group. The NHS has charged primary care groups with responsibility for collectively planning primary care and community health services in their areas, contracting with hospitals and

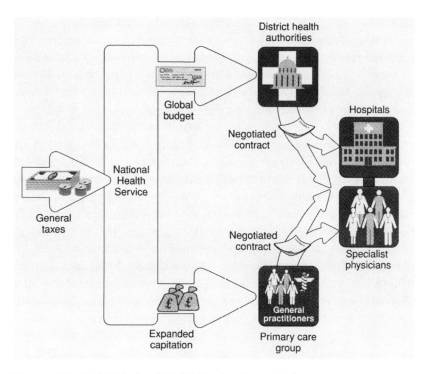

District health
authorities

Global
budget

Hospitals

Negotiated
contract

National
Health
Service

General
taxes

Negotiated
contract

Specialist
physicians

Expanded
capitation

General
practitioners

Primary care
group

Figure 4. The British National Health Service: Recent Reforms

hospital consultants for specialty care, scrutinizing GP practice patterns, and implementing quality improvement activities (Bindman et al., 2001). The average primary care group has about 50 GP members, as well as additional primary care representatives from other professions, and covers a population of about 100,000 enrolled patients (figure 4).

An English primary care group resembles a U.S. independent practice association in some ways. As in an IPA, GPs in the NHS retain ownership of their individual or small group practices while participating in a network of physicians. However, unlike the case in the United States, English GPs are required to participate in the primary care group in their area, and each area has only a single primary care group. Furthermore, while IPAs in the United States tend to have economic survival as their foremost goal and overwhelmingly focus on contract negotiations with managed care plans and processing payments to participating physicians, NHS primary care groups are directed more toward planning for their population's health needs and improving quality of care. For example, primary care groups are expected to select clinical indicators (e.g., treatment of patients with coronary heart disease with aspirin), to review practice patterns for GPs in the group for this indicator, and to develop strategies to improve practices for the indicator. Compared with the complicated arrangements in the U.S., with physicians participating in multiple IPAS and no single network connecting all patients in a geographic region, English primary care groups are truly population-health focused and are accountable for the entire population within a geographic area. Many proponents of primary care groups are hopeful that this organizational structure will help to institutionalize community-oriented primary care and continuous quality improvement, although development of primary care groups is too recent to know whether these organizations will live up to their promise. Critics have expressed concerns that GPs will be ill equipped to handle the managerial responsibilities of community health planning and quality improvement, that GPs will not be granted paid "release time" from their clinical practices to compensate for the greater expectations imposed on them, and that fiscal limitations in the NHS will impede implementation of plans for quality improvement and community care.

Japan

Health Insurance

Akiko Tanino works in the accounting department of the Mazda car company in Tokyo. Like all Mazda employees, she is enrolled in the health insurance plan directly operated by Mazda. Each month, 3.5% of Akiko's salary is deducted from her paycheck and paid to the Mazda health plan. Mazda makes an additional payment to its health plan equivalent to 4.5% of Akiko's salary.

Akiko's father, Takeshi, recently retired after working for many years as an engineer at Mazda. When he retired, his health insurance changed from the Mazda company plan to the citizens health insurance plan administered by the municipal government where he lives. However, Mazda makes payments to the citizens health insurance plan to help pay for the health care costs of the company's retirees. In addition, the citizens health insurance plan requires that Takeshi pay the plan a premium indexed to his income.

Akiko's brother, Kazuo, is a mechanic at a small auto repair shop in Tokyo. He is automatically enrolled in the government managed health insurance plan operated by the Japanese national government. Kazuo and his employer each contribute payments equal to 4.25% of Kazuo's salary to the government plan.

Although Japanese society has a cultural history distinct from the other nations discussed in this chapter, its health care system draws heavily from European and North American traditions. As in Germany, Japan's modern health insurance system is rooted in an employment-linked social insurance program. Japan first legislated mandatory employment-based social insurance for many workers in 1922, building on pre-existing voluntary mutual aid societies. The system was gradually expanded until universal coverage was achieved in 1961 with passage of the National Health Insurance Act. The Japanese insurance system differs from the German model by having different categories of health plans with even more numerous individual plans and less flexibility in choice of plan (figure 5).

Employers with 700 or more employees are required to operate self-insured plans for their employees and dependents, known as "society-managed insurance" plans. Although these plans resemble the German industry-specific sickness funds, each company must operate its own individual health plan. About 1,800 different employer-based plans exist. Eighty-five percent of these society plans are operated by individual companies, with the balance operated as joint plans between two or more employers, although none involves as many companies as the typical German sickness fund. The boards of directors of society plans are composed of 50% employee and 50% employer representatives. Employees and their dependents are required to enroll in their company's society plan, and the employee and employer must contribute a payroll tax to fund the society. Because each plan is self-insured, the payroll tax rate varies depending on the average income and health risk of the company's employees. The payroll tax for the average society plan is 3.7% for the employee and 4.8% for the employer. These society managed insurance plans cover 26% of the Japanese population.

Employees and dependents in companies with fewer than 70 employees are compulsorily enrolled in a single national health insurance plan for small businesses that is operated by the national government. This government managed insurance plan covers 30% of the population. This plan is also primarily financed by payroll taxes, with the federal government

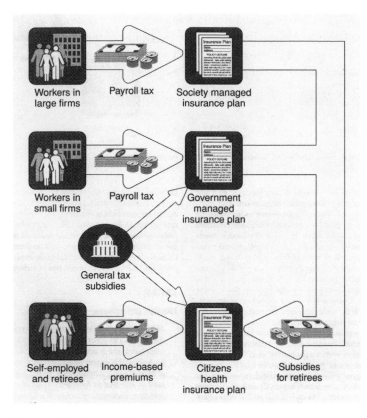

Figure 5. The Japanese Health System

setting a uniform payroll tax of 4.25% for employees and 4.25% for employers. The federal government also uses general tax revenues to subsidize the government managed insurance plan.

Yet a third type of health insurance, the citizens health insurance plan, covers self-employed workers and retirees (35% of the population). Each municipal government in Japan administers a local citizens insurance plan, and levies a compulsory premium to the self-employed workers and retirees in its jurisdiction. In addition, each employer-operated society managed insurance plan and the single government managed insurance plan must contribute payments to the citizens health insurance plan fund to subsidize the costs for retirees. About 40% of the financing for the citizens health insurance program comes from contributions from the society-managed and government-managed insurance plans, making employers liable for a large portion of the costs of their retirees' health care. Additional funds for the citizens health insurance plan come from general tax revenues.

A smattering of smaller insurance programs exist for government employees and other special categories of workers, and resemble the society-managed insurance plans. Persons who become unemployed remain enrolled in their health plan with the payroll tax waived. All plans are required to provide standard comprehensive benefits, including payment for hospital and physician services, prescription drugs, maternity care, and dental care. In addition, in 2000 Japan implemented a new long-term insurance plan, financed by general tax revenues and a new earmarked income tax, that provides comprehensive benefits to disabled adults, including payment for home care, case management, and institutional services.

In summary, Japan—like Germany—builds on an employment-based social insurance model, using additional general tax subsidies to create a universal insurance program. Compared with Germany, the national and local governments in Japan are more involved in directly administering health plans, and a majority of Japanese are covered by government-run plans rather than by employer-managed private plans (Ikegami and Campbell, 1999; Kemporen, 1999).

Medical Care

Takeshi Tanino's knee has been aching for several weeks. He makes an appointment at a clinic operated by an orthopedic surgeon. At the clinic Takeshi has a medical examination, an X-ray of the knee, and is scheduled for regular physical therapy. During the examination the orthopedist notes that Takeshi's blood pressure is high and recommends that Takeshi see an internist at a different clinic about this problem.

Six months later, Takeshi develops a cough and fever. He makes an appointment at the medical clinic of a nearby hospital run by Dr. Suzuki, is diagnosed with pneumonia, and admitted to the medical ward. He is treated with intravenous antibiotics for two weeks, and remains in the hospital for an additional two weeks after completing antibiotics for further intravenous hydration and nursing care.

Health plans place no restrictions on choice of hospital and physician and do not require preauthorization before using medical services. Most medical care is institutionally based in three types of settings: (1) independent clinics, each owned by a physician and staffed by the physician and other employees, with many clinics also having small inpatient wards; (2) small hospitals with inpatient and outpatient departments, owned by a physician with employed physician staff; and (3) larger public and private hospitals with outpatient and inpatient departments and salaried physician staff. Facilities are organized by specialty, with larger hospitals having a wide range of specialties and smaller hospitals and clinics offering a more limited selection of specialty departments. Care is delivered in a specialty-specific manner, with few organizations using a more primary care-oriented, "gatekeeper" model (Smith et al., 1997).

Physician entrepreneurship is a strong element in the organization of health care in Japan. Most clinics and small hospitals are family-owned businesses founded and operated by independent physicians. Unlike clinics in the United States such as the Mayo Clinic and Palo Alto Medical Clinic that began as family-owned institutions but evolved into nonprofit organizations with ownership shared among a larger group of physician partners, most clinics in Japan have remained under the ownership of a single physician, often passed down within a family from one generation to another. Many physicians expanded their clinics to become small hospitals, but the government builds and operates the larger medical centers. Furthermore, the distinction between clinics and hospitals in Japan is not as great as in most nations. Clinics are permitted to operate inpatient beds, and only become classified as hospitals when they have more than 20 beds. About 30% of clinics in Japan have inpatient beds. Virtually all physicians either own clinics and hospitals, or work as employees of a clinic or hospital, and practice only within their single institution. Although many physician-owned clinics and hospitals are modest facilities, others are larger institutions offering a wide array of outpatient and inpatient services featuring the latest biomedical technology, electronic medical records, and automated medication dispensing.

Rates of hospital admission are relatively low in Japan and rates of surgery are only about one-third the rate in the United States (Ikegami and Campbell, 1999). A cultural norm that makes patients reluctant to undergo invasive procedures in part explains the low surgical rate in Japan. When hospitalized, patients remain for an average of 33 days—an unusually long stay compared with the typical length of stay in most developed nations (Kemporen, 1999). Patients are allowed long periods to convalesce while still in the hospital.

Paying Doctors and Hospitals

> One month after returning home from the hospital, Takeshi Tanino develops stomach pain that awakens him several nights. He makes an appointment at a general medical clinic run by Dr. Sansei. Dr. Sansei performs an endoscopy, which reveals gastritis. Dr. Sansei prescribes an H_2 blocker and arranges for Takeshi to return to the clinic every four weeks for the next six months. Takeshi's stomach ache improves after a few days of using the medication. At each follow-up visit, Dr. Sansei questions Takeshi about his symptoms and dispenses a new four-week supply of medications.

Health plans pay both physicians and hospitals on a fee-for-service basis. Government regulates these fees, as well as prices for medications, under the advisement of the Central Social Insurance Medical Council. Physicians, health plans, and the public are represented on the Central Council, with the Japanese Medical Association nominating the physician members. The fee schedule is in many ways the opposite of U.S. fees: In Japan, primary care services tend to command higher fees than do more specialized services such as surgical procedures and imaging studies (Ikegami and Campbell, 1999).

Physicians are permitted to directly dispense medications, not just to prescribe them, and are also allowed to charge a dispensing fee. Many physician visits are brief and, as in the example of Takeshi Tanino's bout of gastritis, focus mainly on renewing medications. People in Japan make 2 1/2 times as many visits to a physician each year as people in the United States, Germany, Canada, and the United Kingdom. The average clinic physician in Japan sees 66 patients each day (Smith et al., 1997).

Cost Control

Health care costs grew rapidly in Japan in the 1970s, rising from 4.0% of GDP in 1970 to 6.0% in 1980. Costs as a proportion of GDP stabilized between 1980 and the mid-1990s, rising only about 1% (from 6.0% to 7.1%) between 1980 and 1995. Two major factors contributed to this stabilization: (1) implementation of more stringent government regulation of fees, and (2) the remarkably rapid growth in the overall Japanese economy, which buffered the effects of health care inflation. However, concerns about increasing health care costs resurfaced in the mid-1990s as Japan entered a sustained economic recession. In addition, the changing demographics of Japan are stressing a health care financing system that relies heavily on payroll taxes. With a plummeting birth rate and the longest life expectancy of any nation in the world, Japan's population is aging faster than that of other developed nations. The proportion of Japanese over age 65 is projected to increase from 10% in 1985 to 26% in 2020. In comparison, the proportion of the U.S. population over age 65 will increase much more modestly, from 12% to 16%, during this same period (Kemporen, 1999).

In 1997, the government imposed greater patient cost sharing in an attempt to contain costs. For most plans, copayments increased from 10% to 20% of all services, although elderly patients were exempted from cost sharing for medications. This policy had minimal impact, experiencing many of the predictable problems of cost sharing. For example, due to concerns about excessive burdens on patients with major illnesses, the monthly limit on out-of-pocket expenditures was capped at about $500; cost sharing thus did little to change the catastrophic medical expenses that account for the majority of health care costs. Currently, the Japanese government and health plans are debating other strategies to contain costs, including shifting to more bundled payment units such as DRGs for hospitals and revising the system of price regulation for drugs. Interestingly, although many nations have shied away from implementing new long-term care insurance programs due to concerns about the high costs associated with an aging population, Japan has met this challenge head on and in 2000 implemented a new national insurance plan for long-term care.

The Japanese Long-Term Care Insurance Plan

Sadako Tanino did what virtually all Japanese women of her generation did. When her parents became disabled with strokes, she cared for them in her home, feeding them, bathing them, and even staying with them in the hospital on occasions when they needed inpatient care. However, when Sadako became disabled by Alzheimer's disease at age 74, there was no one in the family who could care for her in the same way. Both her son and daughter, Kazuo and Akiko, work full time and are raising children. Her husband, Takeshi, is infirm from his own medical problems. Fortunately, Japan enacted a new long-term care insurance plan at just the right time for Sadako. The plan arranges for a physician and geriatric team to evaluate Sadako's functional status and medical condition. The team recommends an adult day health program during the weekdays, supplemented by in-home nursing aide services on the weekends. All these services are covered by the long-term care plan.

The new Japanese long-term care insurance plan integrates medical and social service benefits into a single comprehensive program. All persons aged 65 and over with medical conditions that limit independent living are eligible for services, pending evaluation of their case by a local reviewer. Individuals between the ages of 40 and 65 are eligible only if they have certain types of disabling conditions. Half of the program is financed by income-indexed premiums paid by persons age 40 and over (averaging about $25 per month in 2000), and half is financed through general taxes. In addition, patients pay a copayment of 10% for all services (Kemporen, 1999).

The new plan provides comprehensive benefits, including home visits from nurses, physicians, and allied health personnel, home bathing, medical equipment, day care center services, case management, and institutional care in nursing homes and hospital wards. As with the On Lok program in the United States, one of the primary goals of the new Japanese plan is to maximize opportunities for supported living at home rather than in institutions, and it is hoped that this will simultaneously improve quality and the efficiency of expenditures.

Conclusion

Key issues in evaluating and comparing health care systems are access to care, level of health expenditures, public satisfaction with health care, and the overall quality of care as expressed by the health of the population. We have seen that Germany, Canada, the United Kingdom, and Japan provide universal financial access to health care through government-run or government-mandated programs. We have also seen that these four nations have controlled health care costs more successfully than has the United States (see tables 1 and 2), though all four continue to face challenges in containing their spending.

Table 1. Total Health Expenditures as a Percentage of
Gross Domestic Product (GDP), 1970–1998

	1970	1980	1985	1990	1995	1998
Germany	5.5	7.9	8.7	8.3	10.4	10.6
United Kingdom	4.5	5.8	6.0	6.2	6.9	6.7
Canada	7.2	7.4	8.5	9.5	9.6	9.5
Japan	4.1	6.0	6.2	6.0	7.1	7.6
United States	7.4	9.2	10.5	12.2	13.6	13.6

Source: Anderson and Hussey, 2001.

Table 2. Per Capita Health Spending in U.S. Dollars, 1998

Germany	$2424
United Kingdom	1461
Canada	2312
Japan	1822
United States	4178

In a 1990 survey of 10 nations, Canada ranked first in public satisfaction with the health care system, West Germany ranked third, Japan seventh, the United Kingdom eighth, and the United States came in last (Blendon et al., 1990). During the 1990s, public confidence in the Canadian and German systems declined, although satisfaction remained higher than in the United States (Blendon et al., 1995; Donelan et al., 1999). People in the United States are much more likely than those in Canada and the United Kingdom to report a problem paying their medical bills in the past year. Interestingly, despite the volatility of waiting times as a political issue, only 12% of people surveyed in the United Kingdom reported that they were "very worried" about possible long waits for nonemergency care, a percentage similar to that in the United States (Donelan et al., 1999). A 2000 survey of physicians in different nations found that about a quarter of physicians in Canada and the United Kingdom believe that their health care system "works well and only minor changes are needed," compared with 17% of U.S. physicians (Blendon et al., 2001). German physicians in an earlier survey were the most likely to rate their system highly (Blendon et al., 1993). Similar patterns emerged from a 1999 survey of hospital nurses in these nations. Job dissatisfaction and burnout were highest

Table 3. Health Outcome Measures

	Life Expectancy at Birth			Life Expectancy at Age 60	
	Infant Mortality[1]	Men	Women	Men	Women
Germany	5.3	74.5	80.5	19.0	23.3
United Kingdom	6.2	74.6	79.7	18.8	22.6
Canada	6.3	75.8	81.4	20.0	24.4
Japan	3.8	77.2	84.0	21.0	26.4
United States	8.0	73.9	79.4	19.6	23.1

Source: Anderson and Hussey, 2001.
1. Per 1,000 live births.
Infant mortality data are for 1996; life expectancy data are for 1997 or 1998.

among nurses in the United States, intermediate among those in Canada and the United Kingdom, and lowest among nurses in Germany (Aiken et al., 2001). A majority of nurses in all four nations expressed concerns about inadequate hospital nurse staffing.

Cross-national comparisons of health care quality are treacherous and tend to confuse the impacts of socioeconomic factors and quality of medical care on the health status of the population. But such comparisons can convey rough impressions of whether a health care system is functioning at a reasonable level of quality. From table 3, it is clear that the United States has an infant mortality rate higher than that of Germany, Canada, the United Kingdom, and Japan, with the Japanese rate being the lowest. Japan also has the highest male and female life expectancy rates at birth. The life expectancy rate at age 60 is believed by some observers to measure the impact of medical care, especially its more high-tech component, more than it measures underlying socioeconomic influences. By this standard, the United States moves up in its ranking (Anderson and Hussey, 2001).

Just as epidemiologic studies often derive their most profound insights from comparisons of different populations, research into health services can glean insights from the experience of other nations. As the United States confronts its dual health care problems of limited access and increasing cost, it must look across its borders and overseas to nations who have been more successful in solving those problems.

References

Aaron HJ, Schwartz WB: *The Painful Prescription: Rationing Hospital Care.* The Brookings Institution, 1984.

Aiken LH et al: Nurses' reports on hospital care in five countries. *Health Affairs* 2001;20(3):43.

Anderson GM et al: Use of coronary artery bypass surgery in the United States and Canada. *JAMA* 1993;269:1661.

Anderson G, Hussey PS: Comparing health system performance in OECD countries. *Health Affairs* 2001;20(3):219.

Barer ML, Lomas J, Sanmartin C: Re-minding our Ps and Qs: Medical cost controls in Canada. *Health Affairs* 1996;15(2):216.

Bindman AB, Weiner JP, Majeed A: Primary care groups in the United Kingdom. *Health Affairs* 2001;20(3):132.

Blendon RJ et al: Physicians' perspectives on caring for patients in the United States, Canada, and West Germany. *N Engl J Med* 1993;328:1011.

Blendon RJ et al: Satisfaction with health systems in ten nations. *Health Affairs* 1990;9(2):185.

Blendon RJ et al: Who has the best health care system? A second look. *Health Affairs* 1995;14(4):220.

Blendon RJ et al: Physicians' views on quality of care: a five-country comparison. *Health Affairs* 2001; 20(3):233.

Brown LD, Amelung VE: "Manacled competition:" Market reforms in German health care. *Health Affairs* 1999; 18(3):76.

Coyte PC et al: Waiting times for knee-replacement surgery in the United States and Ontario. *N Engl J Med* 1994; 331:1068.

Donelan K et al: The cost of health care system change: Public discontent in five nations. *Health Affairs* 1999;18(3):206.

Evans RG: Tension, compression, and shear: Directions, stresses, and outcomes of health care cost control. *J Health Polit Policy Law* 1990;15:101.

Evans RG et al: Controlling health expenditures: The Canadian reality. *N Engl J Med* 1989;320:571.

Files A, Murray M: German risk structure compensation: Enhancing equity and effectiveness. *Inquiry* 1995;32:300.

Fuchs VR, Hahn JS: How does Canada do it? *N Engl J Med* 1990; 323:884.

Grumbach K et al: Regionalization of cardiac surgery in the United States and Canada. *JAMA* 1995;274:1282.

Hiatt HH: *America's Health in the Balance.* Harper & Row, 1987.

Iglehart JK: Germany's health care system. *N Engl J Med* 1991;324:503.

Ikegami N, Campbell JC: Health care reform in Japan: The virtues of muddling through. *Health Affairs* 1999;18(3):56.

Katz SJ et al: Comparing use of diagnostic tests in Canadian and U.S. hospitals. *Med Care* 1996a;34:117.

Katz SJ et al: Physician use in Ontario and the United States: The impact of socioeconomic status and health status. *Am J Public Health* 1996b;86:520.

Katz SJ et al: Mental health care use, morbidity, and socioeconomic status in the United States and Ontario. *Inquiry* 1997;34:38.

Kemporen (National Federation of Health Insurance Societies): *Health Insurance and Health Insurance Societies in Japan, 1999*. Kemporen, 1999.

Lister J: Prospects for the National Health Service. *N Engl J Med* 1988;318:1473.

Lomas J et al: Paying physicians in Canada: minding our Ps and Qs. *Health Affairs* 1989;8(1):80.

Maynard A, Bloor K: Introducing a market to the United Kingdom's National Health Service. *N Engl J Med* 1996;334:604.

Menon D: Pharmaceutical cost control in Canada. *Health Affairs* 2001;20(3):92.

Naylor CD: Health care in Canada: incrementalism under fiscal duress. *Health Affairs* 1999;18(3):9.

Payer L: *Medicine and Culture*. Henry Holt, 1988.

Potter C, Porter J: American perceptions of the British National Health Service: Five myths. *J Health Polit Policy Law* 1989;14:341.

Rachlis M, Kushner C: *Second Opinion: What's Wrong with Canada's Health Care System and How to Fix It*. Collins, 1989.

Roemer MI: *National Health Systems of the World*, Vols 1 and 2. Oxford Univ Press, 1993.

Saltman RB (editor): *The International Handbook of Health-Care Systems*. Greenwood Press, 1988.

Schieber GJ, Poullier JP, Greenwald LM: Health spending, delivery, and outcomes in OECD countries. *Health Affairs* 1993;12(2):120.

Sidel VW, Sidel R: *A Healthy State*. Pantheon Books, 1983.

Silberman G et al: Availability and appropriateness of allogenic bone marrow transplantation for chronic myeloid leukemia in 10 countries. *N Engl J Med* 1994;331:1063.

Smith BWH et al: Family medicine in Japan. *Arch Fam Med* 1997;6:59.

Taylor MG: *Insuring National Health Care. The Canadian Experience*. Univ of North Carolina Press, 1990.

Welch WP et al: A detailed comparison of physician services for the elderly in the United States and Canada. *JAMA* 1996;275:1410.

Woolhandler S, Himmelstein DU: The deteriorating administrative efficiency of the U.S. health care system. *N Engl J Med* 1991;324:1253.

Keeping Quality on the Policy Agenda
Elizabeth A. McGlynn and Robert H. Brook

The United States ranks 37th in the world in overall health system performance and 72nd on population health, according to a recent World Health Organization (WHO) report.[1] These rankings are at odds with many Americans' belief that the United States has the best quality of care in the world.[2] Objective information on U.S. health system failures is generally met with a day or two of media flurry and no sustained policy response. By contrast, Congress took immediate steps to identify and correct problems that had led to defective Firestone tires, and the Federal Aviation Administration (FAA) ordered a redesign of faulty rudders on Boeing 737s following a series of reported failures in the 1990s. Policy makers are capable of taking action to protect human life in many other areas, but efforts directed at the health care system remain uncommon. Without sustained public attention to solving the quality deficit problem in health care, little progress will be made.

The Quality of Health Care Is Substandard

How good is quality of care in the United States? We don't really know, but a review of the best scientific literature reveals the following sobering facts.[3] Only half of the population receives needed preventive care; 70% receive recommended care for acute problems, such as colds or stomach pain; and just 60% of those with a chronic illness such as diabetes or hypertension get the care they need. On the other hand, about one-third of the care delivered for acute problems is not needed (for example, antibiotics prescribed for the common cold) and may actually be harmful.

Elizabeth McGlynn and Robert H. Brook, "Keeping Quality on the Policy Agenda," *Health Affairs*, vol. 20, 82–90. © 2001 by Project HOPE—The People-to-People Health Foundation, Inc.

About one-fifth of the care given to persons with chronic conditions is also unnecessary and possibly harmful. Given the public outcry over a few deaths from bad tires, the lack of public outrage over thousands of preventable deaths in medicine is astounding.

Serious deficits are also manifest in how skillfully care is delivered. Coronary angiography is an invasive test used to diagnose cardiac disease and determine what treatment is appropriate for a patient. Analysis of a random sample of angiographies performed in one state showed that only half of the tests were done competently enough to be accurately interpreted.[4] When the tests were reread by a group of expert cardiologists, one-quarter of patients determined by the original reading to have the most severe disease did not have it. Six percent of persons who were told that their test results were not severely abnormal actually had severely abnormal results. One-third of persons whose bypass surgery was considered necessary or appropriate based on the original interpretation of the angiography results underwent surgery that was of uncertain benefit or inappropriate based on the gold-standard review. Nearly 1.3 million coronary angiographies were performed in 1998 nationally. If the results of this study held nationally, nearly 650,000 tests would be difficult to interpret accurately; at $12,450 per test, that is more than $8 billion in wasted expense.

Countless other examples show that medicine as practiced in the United States today is dangerous. The Institute of Medicine recently estimated that as many as 98,000 people may die in any given year from medical errors.[5] Although stories on errors in medicine continue to appear in the media, serious action to improve the situation has yet to emerge.

Deficits in quality of care are not unique to the United States. A summary of the international literature showed that only about half of what is recommended in medicine gets done.[6] Studies of the appropriateness of various diagnostic and therapeutic surgical procedures in the United Kingdom, Canada, Israel, and Sweden show similar results to those in the United States.[7]

Such statistics point to health care systems that pose real and potential threats to human life far greater than those from defective tires or airplane rudders. Deficits in quality have been noted consistently throughout the past three or four decades, despite changes in how services are paid for (for example, prospective payment under Medicare) or delivered (managed care). Quality deficits are also found in countries with very different organizational and financial structures. Fixing quality requires a fundamentally different policy approach than either increasing or reducing expenditures.

Why Is It So Difficult to Sustain Public Interest?

The message that there is a problem with the quality of health care around the world is not a new one. Given that poor quality affects whether and how well people live, why is it so difficult to sustain public interest in this problem? We provide several reasons that underscore how the health care system differs from other economic sectors. Strategies to address these barriers should be useful for improving quality in the United States and internationally.

Diffuse Responsibility

When a problem with the processes or outcomes of care is identified, no single or large manufacturer is to blame—no Firestone or Boeing. Research has shown that persons undergoing coronary artery bypass graft surgery have a variable likelihood of survival after the procedure.[8] However, to motivate improved surgical care, problems must be identified and solutions developed in each of thousands of hospitals. There is rarely a credible threat that poor-quality providers will be driven out of business or even suffer a significant loss of revenue.

The Health Care Financing Administration (HCFA) tried in the mid-1980s to create an environment of accountability by developing standardized reports on whether the death rate in each hospital was what one might expect given how sick the patients were at admission. These mortality reports were discontinued in 1993 primarily for political reasons, but they inspired the development of some local organizations (for example, the Northern New England Cardiovascular Disease Study Group) dedicated to improving care. Although some of these efforts have been successful, few such examples exist nationally. Even the Peer Review Organization (PRO) program, which has been overseeing quality in the Medicare program since 1986, has not solved the problem of substandard care.[9]

Cognitive Dissonance

Most people assume that their own doctor is excellent and that any problems identified by researchers, accreditors, the media, or malpractice lawyers affect someone else. Most doctors believe that they deliver care consistent with guidelines and standards. But if the public and the medical profession do not acknowledge that suboptimal care is delivered throughout the medical care system and that significant reengineering is essential, then thousands more lives will be needlessly lost.

Reports on medical errors have come closest in recent times to breaking through this cognitive dissonance. We need to find ways to use the dialogue that has begun around errors to promote a shared understanding of the quality problem without fundamentally undermining trust in the medical care system.

Outmoded System Design

The U.S. health care system is a technological anomaly. We have made amazing advances in the availability of diagnostic machines, chemicals to treat or cure illnesses, and microsurgical techniques to repair the ravages of disease or injury. Yet most physicians and hospitals rely on barely legible, handwritten notes to track what is done to a patient and how the patient responds.

Doctors also are expected to maintain in their individual memories the appropriate approaches to diagnosing and treating a wide variety of diseases as they are manifest in human beings of radically different designs (age, race, height, weight, other health problems). By contrast, airline pilots are only allowed to fly one type of airplane and rely on extensive checklists and computer monitoring to ensure its safe operation. Nonetheless, we are surprised when physicians, using systems from the 19th century, and subject to the limitations of being human, fall well short of perfection.

The medical establishment has actively dismissed attempts to introduce systems principles into medical care. Physicians dismiss "cookbook" medical practice as if consistent delivery of known practices is necessarily a bad thing. In many other areas of consumable goods and services, consumers expect to get the same thing (such as a Big Mac or local currency from an automated teller machine anywhere in the world), at the same level of quality, no matter where they are. In medicine, the focus on individually tailored services means that if one has a heart attack, survival is dependent on whether the hospital used—usually the closest one—consistently uses appropriate and timely diagnostic and therapeutic procedures.

Much of the research on quality looks retrospectively at whether care already delivered is consistent with standards. Although these methods are useful for documenting the nature of the problem, they do not offer a solution. We cannot recall defective medical care the way we can recall a defective car. Systems must be in place to guide doctors' actions while the patient is being seen or to bring patients in for routine monitoring.

Information Void

We lack basic, objective information on how well the health system is functioning and what would make it function better. There is no national tracking system for identifying defects and correcting them before someone dies. There are few early warning systems to identify problems before they become widespread. There are no systems in place for ensuring that best practices are consistently implemented. There is almost no systematic information on what reengineering strategies are likely to work on a large scale. Many small projects (including many of the PRO projects) done in one state, one health system, or one hospital have demonstrated that improvement is possible. These individual projects (many of which are never published) have not led to any generalized knowledge of what changes are necessary to improve quality. Randomized trials in this area are rare but can add much to our understanding of generalizable quality improvement techniques.[10]

The Tendency to Shoot the Messenger

Finally, a common response to objective quality-performance results is to insist that the data are inaccurate and do not reflect what is really happening in any particular hospital or doctor's office. This attitude is part of what led to the demise of the HCFA mortality reports. Doctors and system administrators are not only reluctant to use information, they are often reluctant to participate in efforts to obtain good information about performance. This shoot-the-messenger attitude means that more energy is devoted to undermining the findings than to formulating and implementing solutions.

Is Change Hopeless, or Can We Make Progress?

The authors of this essay, perhaps eternal optimists, remain hopeful that change is possible. Because the problem is complex and the solutions require innovative strategies, we must generate sustained public interest to improve quality. Patience and perseverance will be essential, as will cooperation between the private and public sectors. We would like to give an outline of the exact interventions that would work best, but this knowledge does not exist. Leadership is the necessary first step.

Create Quality Champions

Fundamentally, we need a "war on poor quality" that has the same level of public commitment as the war on cancer or the campaign to put a man on the moon. We believe that the subsequent funding of needed research in response to this declaration of war will lead to the development of specific strategies that should be followed. Both the private and public sectors will have to demand a complete overhaul of medical practice, and implementing such change will necessitate leadership from clinicians and a vigilant constituency.

Advocacy organizations have been successful in raising funds for research related to curing specific diseases such as human immunodeficiency virus (HIV) or breast cancer. If such groups added to their mission pressure on health systems and public and private purchasers to pay only for high-quality care that is consistent with best practices, great progress could be made. These advocacy organizations could be champions who would put quality first and insist on design changes that ensure that the health care system gets the fundamentals right.

Medicare could similarly become a quality champion by setting higher standards for public reporting on quality. HCFA does require that managed care plans report data on measures in the Health Plan Employer Data and Information Set (HEDIS). The National Committee for Quality Assurance (NCQA) has demonstrated that managed care plans publicly reporting HEDIS data for three consecutive years have higher quality than plans that do not make data available.[11] But we can no longer tolerate the lack of information on performance in the non–managed care sector.

Develop a Functional Information System

Second, health care professionals and organizations need to embrace computer technologies that can be used to receive and transmit information. The private sector should lead the way by making investment in such systems an allowable expense in calculating health insurance premiums.

The government should undertake an evaluation of tax incentives that might further spur the adoption of computer technologies in office-based medical practice. No serious advances in quality of care can be made without a functioning, computer-based information system. Computerized order-entry systems used in hospitals have been shown to reduce adverse events associated with errors in the prescribing and administering of medications.[12]

Right now, nobody is penalized financially for failing to adopt computerized clinical management systems. Regulators and purchasers should use every available tool to provide such a disincentive. Adequate clinical management hardware and software could become a condition of licensure, contracting, malpractice insurance policies, and reimbursement. Although these demands could not be made overnight, compliance within five years would be more than reasonable in the current environment.

Routinely Monitor and Report on Performance

Third, an independent group should routinely compile information into a national report on whether average levels of and variation in quality are increasing or decreasing. There have been scattered attempts to do this, including an effort mandated by Congress, but the amount of funding allocated to these efforts has been grossly inadequate. The New York State Cardiac Reporting System offers an example of the benefits to be had from public reporting. Risk-adjusted mortality rates following bypass surgery have declined significantly in the state since the reporting system was introduced.[13]

To motivate change, public reports on communities, hospitals, health systems, and providers must also be available. Communities could compete to provide the best care to their citizens: If you have a heart attack in Paris, London, or Los Angeles, in which city are you most likely to survive? Families regularly make relocation decisions based on the quality of schools in any area; they might choose to factor quality of medical care into the equation as well.

Ensure Adequate Funding for Quality Measurement

To make all of this work, sustained investments must be made in the tools that are used to set standards, promulgate current and scientifically valid measures for monitoring, provide consistent information to physicians on best practices, make information easily accessible to decision makers, and so on. This is not a trivial enterprise.

Developing guidelines for care is difficult and expensive, and it requires the highest level of scientific integrity. If guidelines are promulgated by individuals without much support, they will be done carelessly and will be (properly) ignored. If guidelines are issued by those who stand to benefit financially, they will be suspect and fail to attract necessary consensus. The Agency for Healthcare Research and Quality (AHRQ) should have as its primary mission improving quality of care through facilitating use of information systems, developing guidelines and other standards of practice, updating and improving quality measurement tools, producing data for national reports on quality, and developing a strategic plan for quality improvement. This ambitious and essential undertaking will require a few billion dollars of new money each year. This amount pales in comparison with total spending on health care (more than $1 trillion), the size of the proposed tax cut ($1.6 trillion), and the budget of the National Institutes of Health ($19 billion in 2001).[14] AHRQ will have to be insulated from political forces that have previously limited its ability to provide strong leadership.

Where might these steps take us by the year 2010? They could mean that people, especially when they required urgent care, would not have to worry about where they go for care. Patients and their families might not need to be warned, as they are today, that they should carefully monitor what medical services they do and do not receive because their inattention might result in serious problems. The science that the nation spent so much public and private money developing could produce its promised benefits. Waste could be eliminated so that all Americans, not just those who have health insurance, could get the care they need.

These achievements are within our grasp. We spend more money on health care than any country in the world; one of every seven dollars spent in this country goes to medical care.[15] We have sophisticated physicians and social scientists. But we lack the will to reengineer our own health system.

Leadership for this reengineering will have to come from both government and the private sector. The government role is particularly critical, something that has been recognized in all other Western nations except the United States. Reengineering the health care system will be complicated by the fact that we cannot shut down the system and import our health care while we slowly redesign processes and plants. We must develop an incentive structure that promotes reengineering while enabling us to operate a system that is providing care to patients.

We must find a way to keep quality of care at the top of the health policy agenda. After providing insurance to all Americans, there is no issue of equal importance.

Notes

1   World Health Organization, *The World Health Report 2000: Health Systems—Improving Performance* (Geneva: WHO, 2000).
2   R.J. Blendon, M. Kim, and J.M. Benson, "The Public versus the World Health Organization on Health System Performance," *Health Affairs* (May–June 2001):10–20.
3   M.A. Schuster, E.A. McGlynn, and R.H. Brook, "How Good Is the Quality of Health Care in the United States?" *Milbank Quarterly* 76, no. 4 (1998):517–563.
4   L.L. Leape et al., "Effect of Variability in the Interpretation of Coronary Angiograms on the Appropriateness of Use of Coronary Revascularization Procedures," *American Heart Journal* 139, no. 1, part 1 (2000):106–113.
5   Institute of Medicine, *To Err Is Human: Building a Safer Health System* (Washington: National Academy Press, 1999).
6   J.M. Grimshaw and I.T. Russell, "Effect of Clinical Guidelines on Medical Practice: A Systematic Review of Rigorous Evaluations," *Lancet* 342, no. 8883 (1993):1317–1322.
7   D. Gray et al., "Audit of Coronary Angiography and Bypass Surgery," *Lancet* 335, no. 8701 (1990): 1317–1320; E.A. McGlynn et al., "A Comparison of the Appropriateness of Coronary Angiography and Coronary Artery Bypass Graft Surgery between Canada and New York State," *Journal of the American Medical Association* 272, no. 12 (1994):934–940; D. Pilpel et al., "Regional Differences in Appropriateness of Cholecystectomy in a Prepaid Health Insurance System," *Public Health Review* 20, no. 1–2 (1992–1993):61–74; and S.J. Bernstein et al., "Appropriateness of Referral of Coronary Angiography Patients in Sweden: SECOR/SBU Project Group," *Heart* 81, no. 5 (1999):470–477.
8   G.T. O'Connor et al., "A Regional Prospective Study of In-Hospital Mortality Associated with Coronary Artery Bypass Grafting: The Northern New England Cardiovascular Disease Study Group," *Journal of the American Medical Association* 266, no. 6 (1991):803–809; H.S.Luft and P.S. Romano, "Chance, Continuity, and Change in Hospital Mortality Rates: Coronary Artery Bypass Graft Patients in California Hospitals, 1983 to 1989," *Journal of the American Medical Association* 270, no. 3 (1993):331–337; E.L. Hannan et al., "Improving the Outcomes of Coronary Artery Bypass Surgery in New York State," *Journal of the American Medical Association* 271, no. 10 (1994):761–766; and W.A. Ghali et al., "Coronary Artery Bypass Grafting in Canada: Hospital Mortality Rates, 1992–1995," *Canadian Medical Association Journal* 159, no. 8 (1998):926–930.
9   S.F. Jencks et al., "Quality of Medical Care Delivered to Medicare Beneficiaries: A Profile at State and National Levels," *Journal of the American Medical Association* 284, no. 13 (2000):1670–1676.
10 K.B. Wells et al., "Impact of Disseminating Quality Improvement Programs for Depression in Managed Primary Care: A Randomized Controlled Trial," *Journal of the American Medical Association* 283, no. 2 (2000):212–220.

11   National Committee for Quality Assurance, *The State of Managed Care Quality* (Washington: NCQA, 1999).

12   D.W. Bates et al., "Effect of Computerized Physician Order Entry and a Team Intervention on Prevention of Serious Medication Errors," *Journal of the American Medical Association* 280, no. 15 (1998):1311–1316.

13   Hannan et al., "Improving the Outcomes of Coronary Artery Bypass Surgery."

14   C.A. Cowan et al., "National Health Expenditures, 1998," *Health Care Financing Review* 21, no. 2 (1999):165–210; G. Kessler and E. Pianin, "Bush Tax Cut Faces Spending Pressures," *Washington Post,* 25 January 2001, A1; and National Institutes of Health Press Briefing on FY 2001 President's Budget, ⟨www4.od.nih.gov/ofm/budget/fy2001pressbrief ing.htm⟩ (15 March 2001).

15   Selected national health accounts indicators for all World Health Organization member states, estimates for 1997, Statistical Annex, Table 8 ⟨www.who.int/whr/2000/en/report.htm⟩ (15 March 2001); and Cowan et al., "National Health Expenditures, 1998."

What's Ahead for Health Insurance in the United States?
Victor R. Fuchs

The announcement that most of the nation's biggest insurers—Aetna, CIGNA, Humana, the United Health Group, and Wellpoint Health Network—will be introducing a new kind of health plan during the next year or two signals the beginning of a new era in health insurance in the United States.[1] These plans feature a complicated menu of premiums, copayments, and deductibles that will add impetus to the trend of employers' offering a defined contribution for health benefits. Each employee will get a fixed amount of money to spend as he or she sees fit and will use the Internet to "shop" for medical care. The plans will encourage the use of medical savings accounts in combination with catastrophic-illness insurance to cover expenditures that exceed a large deductible. One of their major effects will be to shift the burden of health care costs from employees who use little care to those who use more. Thus, the new plans will be another nail in the coffin of health insurance as a form of social insurance.

The Erosion of Social Insurance

At its inception, the health insurance system in the United States was very much a social enterprise. Nonprofit insurance companies such as Blue Cross and Blue Shield and the Kaiser Permanente Health Plan charged the same premium for everyone in a community, so that the young and the healthy subsidized the old and the sick. Hospitals also played a part in cross-subsidization by not allocating charges fully to the patients who made the greatest use of the hospital's resources. Many physicians also contributed to the implicit social insurance by providing care to sick poor persons at lower fees or completely free of charge.

This system of social insurance began to erode when private health insurance companies entered the market and instituted policies that departed from the use of community-wide premiums. They used the actuarial approach to insurance, charging lower premiums for groups that were expected to use health care services less. This practice enabled them to "skim the cream" off the top of the health insurance market, and it drove up costs for any plan that tried to continue to set the same premium for everyone. Eventually, standard, community-wide premiums virtually disappeared. Today, most large employers and many medium-size ones are self-insured; they contract with insurance companies for administrative services only. Other employers are typically "experience-rated": their premiums are periodically adjusted to take account of the health care expenditures for their employees during the previous period. Contracts for managed care also erode social insurance by reducing or eliminating the ability of hospitals and physicians to act as agents of redistribution through the cross-subsidization of patients.

Self-insurance, experience rating, and the spread of managed care have ended the subsidization of health care across employers. But there is still cross-subsidization within individual organizations. The new health plans will erode this type of subsidization as well. Once it does so, the only remaining rationale for employment-based health insurance will be the outdated, inequitable tax law that allows employers to deduct their contributions to health insurance and allows employees not to include the value of their health benefits in their taxable income.

Advantages and Disadvantages of the New Plans

Advocates of the new plans claim that the actuarial approach to health insurance is more efficient and more equitable than the social insurance model. They assert that the use of medical care is affected by personal behavior and choice. If costs to individual persons vary with use, they will have an incentive to choose healthier behavior and to make more cost-conscious decisions about care for any given health condition. If cigarette smokers have to spend more for care, the argument goes, they may stop smoking. And if they do not, many assert, it is only fair that smokers bear the cost of their unhealthy habit.

Out-of-pocket payments do give patients an incentive to use less care; whether they are able to make appropriate choices is much more doubtful. The RAND Health Insurance Experience showed that patients with less insurance used less care, but the proportion of care that experts deemed "appropriate" did not vary with the extent of insurance coverage.[2]

Another alleged advantage of the new plans is that they will offer employees more choice and greater flexibility in how they use their health benefits. But choice will turn out to be a two-edged sword. It is a fundamental principle of health insurance that more choice implies more adverse selection—that is, it draws a greater proportion of enrollees with potentially costly health care needs. Insured women who are expecting to have a baby could choose a plan with generous maternity benefits. Patients with diabetes could choose a plan that offers better coverage for chronic care. Adverse selection is the Achilles heel of any voluntary insurance plan.

Moreover, insurance companies, ever on the lookout for a competitive edge, could design benefits packages that would appeal to persons who are basically healthy and discourage enrollment by those who are not. Successful health maintenance organizations have achieved profitability primarily by shrewd underwriting, not by arranging for more efficient delivery of care. New developments in genetic testing and information technology could potentially enhance the ability of insurance companies to practice selective underwriting.

The principal motivation behind the new plans, as behind most health insurance innovations of the past quarter-century, is to slow the rate of growth of health care expenditures. To this end, high hopes are resting on large deductibles combined with catastrophic-illness insurance. These hopes are not likely to be realized.

Problems with Reliance on Catastrophic-Illness Insurance

Medical savings accounts are supposed to make individual patients pay the full price of their care until they exhaust their deductible and the catastrophic-illness insurance kicks in. All use after that point is free from the point of view of the patient. One problem with this approach is that in any given year, a very large fraction of expenditures are accounted for by a very small proportion of patients—patients whose health care costs will exceed any reasonable deductible. It has been estimated that more than half of all expenditures for acute care are accounted for by only 5% of the population.[3]

Moreover, the current distribution of annual expenditures below and above the amount of the deductible exaggerates the proportion of use that will be "price-sensitive" for two reasons. First, a considerable amount of care is elective with respect to timing. Persons who have exceeded their deductible have a great incentive to undergo all the tests and other procedures that they are contemplating in the same year, because there will be no cost to them. If the use of medical savings accounts and catastrophic-illness insurance becomes widespread, the proportion of the nation's total expenditure that is above the amount of the deductible will be much greater than that projected on the basis of current patterns of use of health care. Second, even for those who have not yet exceeded their deductible but expect to do so before the end of the year, any particular test, visit, or procedure will effectively be free, because their total outlay (the deductible) will be the same regardless of whether or not they have the test.

Another problem with the approach of requiring a large deductible is that a deductible that might be reasonable for an employee earning $100,000 per year would be a strain for one earning $50,000 and out of reach for a worker earning $25,000 per year. If the solution is to vary the deductible with income, other problems will arise. If the choice of a deductible is the enrollee's and can be changed during the yearly open-enrollment period, then the potential for adverse selection is great. If the deductible is set according to income by the employer or by law, the administrative problems will be huge. Will the deductible be based on current income or income during the previous year? If the former, the appropriate deductible will not be known until the year is over. If the latter, a decrease in income may make the deductible too large. Will the deductible be based on the employee's wages or on the total household income? The latter is more appropriate, but it is more difficult to determine. How will patients (or providers) know whether the deductible has been exceeded, given that some bills come in many months after the date of care? Regardless of how these questions are answered, it will be expensive to monitor the program.

Also, large deductibles backed up by catastrophic-illness insurance tend to discourage the use of preventive care and encourage expensive high-technology interventions for those who are very ill. Preventive care will often not be covered by catastrophic-illness insurance; thus, the cost to the patient will discourage use. Care for the very ill will usually be covered by the catastrophic-illness insurance. The bias in insurance coverage will bias the development and marketing efforts of drug companies and other suppliers of medical goods and services away from innovations in preventive care.

Finally, there is the question of values. Should health insurance be organized on the same principles as automobile or homeowner's insurance? When drivers with good safety records or homeowners who install smoke detectors are charged less for their automobile or homeowner's insurance, most people see the system as fair and conducive to socially desirable behavior. But the actuarial model applied to health care conflicts with a sense of justice and collective responsibility: it attacks a core element of what it means to be a society. In the long run, the extreme actuarial approach will probably be rejected by the people of the United States as an unsatisfactory way of providing basic health care of all.

The Reemergence of Social Insurance

The case for the fairness of the social-insurance model will be strengthened as people realize that most health problems have, at least in part, a genetic basis. The case for the model's efficiency will benefit from recognition that employment-based insurance has high administrative costs but provides no advantages to society as a whole. The desire to exert more direct control over increasing expenditures will provide an additional reason to introduce some form of national health insurance.

The timing of such a change, however, will depend largely on factors external to health care. Major changes in health policy are political acts undertaken for political purposes. The political nature of such changes was apparent when Bismarck introduced national health insurance to the new German state in the 19th century. It was apparent when England adopted national health insurance after World War II; and it will be apparent in the United States as well. National health insurance will probably come to the United States after a major change in the political climate— the kind of change that often accompanies a war, a depression, or large-scale civil unrest. Until then, the chief effect of the new plans will be to make young and healthy workers better off at the expense of their older, sicker colleagues.

Notes

1 M. Freudenheim. A new health plan may raise expenses for sickest workers. *New York Times*, December 5, 2001: A1.

2 A. L. Siu, F. A. Sonnenberg, W. G. Manning, et al. Inappropriate use of hospitals in a randomized trial of health insurance plans. *New England Journal of Medicine* 315 (1986): 1259–66.

3 H. J. Aaron. Health care reform: the clash of goals, facts, and ideology. In *Individual and social responsibility: child care, education, medical care, and long-term care in America,* ed. V. R. Fuchs, 107–35. Chicago: University of Chicago Press, 1996.

Luxury Primary Care—
Market Innovation or Threat to Access?
Troyen A. Brennan

Primary care practitioners in several states have recently decided to restructure their practices in a way that enables them to see a much smaller number of patients and to spend more time with the ones they do see. Patients enrolled in these practices, referred to as "luxury primary care," pay an annual fee to the practice. In return for this annual fee, they can expect certain amenities that are not currently part of primary care, such as access to their physicians 24 hours a day, 7 days a week, using cell phones or prompt paging devices.[1] When they see their primary care physicians, they can expect up to an hour-long visit. The primary care provider is no longer under pressure to see as many patients as possible each day, because the up-front fee paid by the patient changes the financial structure of the practice. Physicians can even accompany their patients on visits to specialists or to the hospital.

Many physicians are enthusiastic about this new approach because it allows them to take more time in providing care for individual patients. Many patients who dislike the rapid pace and tight schedules that have become characteristic of primary care in the United States are also attracted to this model.[2]

However, some physicians have criticized this approach to primary care, pointing out that only the wealthy can afford such amenities and that physicians should not be catering to wealthy patients. They also claim that these practices are unethical, because patients who cannot afford to pay the annual fee are not allowed into the practice, and long-standing ties with such patients may be severed, disrupting the continuity of care.[3] Some policy analysts wonder whether insurance rules will permit physicians to collect annual fees while they are being reimbursed by insurers for office visits and procedures.[1] In this essay, I examine the features of luxury primary care practices and also discuss the legal and ethical issues that arise with such practices.

Market Innovation

The great debate in health policy over the past two decades has been the proper role of the market in medical care.[4,5] Traditionally, there was no firmly established set of market incentives in medical care. Such incentives were crowded out by professional values and a peculiar set of financial relationships among patients, insurers, and physicians.[6] However, the federal government and many states have introduced market-based reforms in an effort to control costs.

Luxury primary care is an excellent example of a market innovation that serves the interests of both consumers (patients) and suppliers (physicians). The consumers in this case are patients who wish to pay extra for certain amenities that are currently unavailable in primary care. A primary care practice requires a substantial flow of patients in order to be financially viable.[7] Given the relatively low level of reimbursement for a standard office visit and the diminishing amount of money available for the provision of ancillary testing and services, most primary care providers are expected to handle 4,000 or more visits per year. With approximately 240 workdays in a given year, primary care providers must therefore see approximately 20 patients a day. In a standard practice, the time allotted for each visit is 15 minutes for an established patient and 25 minutes for a new patient. Surveys of patients and doctors suggest that they are very unhappy with the amount of time allotted for visits,[8,9] even though empirical research suggests that the time has remained relatively constant over the past decade.[10]

The majority of American citizens have health insurance supplied by their employers, and a substantial minority may have some additional dollars to commit to health care. Thus, there may be a market for practices in which physicians spend more time with patients in return for an annual fee, especially if the fee is only a supplemental payment, with the rest of the costs of health care covered by the patient's health insurance.

Most luxury primary care practices fit this model, although the details vary. The patient usually pays a set fee for entry into the practice.[1] The fee ranges from $1,000 to $20,000 annually but in most cases is at the lower end of the range. The Dare Center in Seattle, for example, charges an annual fee of $3,000.[11] Each physician provides care for 200 to 300 patients (compared with approximately 1,200 to 1,600 patients in many standard primary care practices). The resulting gross revenue per physician—approximately $600,000—is greater than that in a highly efficient primary care practice with the requisite 4,000 visits per year. Insurance reimbursements are therefore merely supplementary dollars rather than the lifeblood of the luxury primary care practice.

With substantial revenues from the annual fees that patients pay, physicians in luxury primary care practices can see fewer patients per day and have time for other activities, such as accompanying patients on visits to specialists. Since the average patient visits a primary care physician two to five times per year, a physician providing care for 200 to 300 patients would have a total of 1,500 or fewer visits. In another model, the annual fee is much lower, and the physicians see a larger number of patients. For example, MDVIP of Boca Raton, Florida, charges $1,500 annually. MDVIP emphasizes preventive care through regular physical examinations and wellness planning, as well as on-line health information.

Many providers will find this approach to primary care practice attractive. Almost all primary care physicians dislike the need to see patients at a rapid pace all day long in order to ensure the financial viability of the practice. They generally do not understand why reimbursement patterns cannot be changed so that such a high volume of visits is not required.[12]

The luxury style of practice may well represent a return to what many providers consider the old days, when physicians had ample time to spend with patients and could really undertake the ethical responsibility to put the patient's welfare above everything else. In addition, the small errors that can occur with rapid-fire primary care may be reduced with luxury primary care, resulting in better care for patients.[13] Certainly, from a professional viewpoint, this new approach promises a much richer and more satisfying practice. Thus, at first blush, luxury primary care appears to be the kind of market innovation that both physicians and patients would welcome.

Although the proponents of luxury primary care acknowledge that not all patients can afford to pay for such care, they argue that there are luxuries unavailable to many people in all sectors of our economy. The analogy to education is especially telling. Many children are educated in public schools, but a substantial minority of children attend private schools that cost much more per year than a luxury primary care practice would. Neither the administrators of such schools nor the parents of the children who attend them have qualms about the fact that not all parents can afford to give their children a private education. Moreover, the teachers enjoy the same professional rewards as teachers in public schools. Like private education, luxury primary care is simply a response to a market need.

The Expectations of Insurers

As noted above, one of the assumptions of luxury primary care is that patients retain their health insurance. Although health insurance is not critical to the operation of the luxury primary care practice, since patients pay an additional premium, reimbursements from insurers for visits reduce the amount that the practice must charge for the luxury premium. More important, health insurance is still relied on to cover the costs of hospitalization, specialty care, and other sorts of care that patients may need. In effect, patients leave the luxury practice whenever they are hospitalized or receive care from a specialist.

Traditionally, insurance arrangements have not entailed an expectation that the insurance payment alone would be sufficient to cover the cost of care provided to the patient. Almost every form of health insurance has a set of copayments or deductibles for which the patient is liable.[14] In addition, some services are not covered. Insurers essentially treat uncovered services, such as cosmetic plastic surgery, as luxury items. Therefore, one might expect that traditional insurance plans would easily accommodate luxury primary care.

However, the situation is not that simple. There are certain insurance arrangements in which the expectation is that the payment provided by the insurer is sufficient to cover the cost of the care. These arrangements prohibit so-called balance billing (the practice of billing the patient for the portion of the physician's fee that is not covered by the insurance payment).[15] Balance billing used to be quite prevalent but has become less so in the past two decades.[15]

Medicare in particular has been hostile to balance billing. At one time, balance billing of Medicare beneficiaries was the norm, and physicians could bill patients for the portion of fees Medicare did not cover. To counteract this practice, Medicare has gradually introduced penalties for physicians who do not accept the Medicare reimbursement as full payment, and today most physicians are not allowed to bill patients for the balance.[16]

Medicare has pursued this policy for a number of reasons. First, Medicare wants to keep health care costs for its beneficiaries under control. In addition, Medicare has strived to create what it believes to be an adequate payment system, a perception that would be undermined if balance billing were allowed.

In many states, commercial insurers and Medicaid programs have followed Medicare's lead. For example, in Massachusetts, the state-regulated Blue Cross program successfully lobbied for a ban on balance billing.[17] The legislature also imposed balance-billing bans for Medicaid. Many commercial insurers include a prohibition of balance billing in their terms of participation for individual physicians. Thus, providers are often not able to obtain their usual and customary fees by charging patients the balance for a service once the insurer has paid its share.

It follows that some insurers might balk at the luxury tax for primary care, for several reasons. First, they may think it is unfair for a patient who pays an insurance premium to be charged an additional premium, even if it is the patient's choice to do so. More likely, insurers may fear that patients who join luxury practices will expect not only highly personal care but also luxurious care in terms of diagnostic and therapeutic procedures. In addition, typical arrangements for ensuring that primary care providers act as gatekeepers, such as capitation mechanisms and the withholding of fees, will probably not be very effective if the primary care provider's main source of income is the luxury premium. Insurers are therefore concerned that luxury primary care will result in high rates of use of specialty services, with the patients in these practices essentially having a free ride on other patients' premiums.

Insurers are definitely studying luxury primary care but have not yet decided how to proceed. None of those I contacted wanted to be on the record. The Center for Medicare and Medicaid Services is simply watching the development of these practices, in effect giving physicians at least a yellow light, if not a green light, to proceed.[1] An executive of a managed care company expressed doubt that his company would contract with luxury care providers, since the annual fee that they charge patients would be viewed as an access fee, which is prohibited.

From the standpoint of market choice and product innovation, it may seem surprising that there are professional or ethical questions about luxury primary care. Physicians providing such care can make a reasonable argument that they are able to provide their patients with the time and effort that every patient should receive.

Nevertheless, there are ethical issues. The first concerns the transition to a luxury practice. Most physicians who are interested in providing luxury primary care are going to make the leap once they know that there is adequate demand for it in their own practice. That means that most practitioners will be making the move from a fully staffed, traditional primary care practice to the new practice. To do so, they must rid themselves of patients who do not wish or cannot afford to pay the luxury tax. Opponents of luxury care argue that these patients will be abandoned and that their care will suffer.

Medical ethics prohibits physicians from abandoning sick patients. This prohibition is supported by the common law, which allows patients, within the context of an established relationship with a physician, to sue the physician for inappropriately refusing to provide further care.[18] But both medical ethics and the common law allow physicians to terminate their relationships with patients. If a patient is receiving treatment for an acute disorder, the physician must continue to provide care.[19] In the case of a patient with an acute problem that has been managed, however, or a patient who is relatively healthy, the relationship can be terminated by finding another physician to provide care for the patient. Therefore, as long as practitioners who make the transition to luxury care do so carefully, by winnowing down their practice and providing patients with referrals to other physicians, there should be no serious ethical or legal impediments.[20] MDVIP, for example, assists doctors with the transition by setting up a call center for patients.

Apart from the prohibition of abandonment, traditional medical ethics is rather poorly equipped to address issues related to luxury primary care. Ethical standards in medicine have focused on the physician's commitment to individual patients and have not addressed broader financial and political issues.[4] Slowly, however, views on these issues have evolved, and over the past 15 years, many have argued that resources—and limits on resources—have to play an important part in medical ethics.[21,22] Energized by debates on managed care, most ethicists now agree that the financial structure of health care is an important subject for ethical consideration.[23] Access to health care, in particular, is a salient ethical issue.[24]

Opponents of luxury primary care argue that its effect on access is the main problem. If almost all primary care physicians charged luxury fees before providing care for patients, then access to health care would certainly be affected. Luxury primary care would have a regressive effect on the health care system, reducing access.

Advocates of luxury primary care counter that they are simply filling a small niche. They point out that at the premium level required for a true luxury practice, relatively few patients will be interested in paying for such care and that it thus does not pose a threat to health care access in general.

Since professional ethics is a matter of reasoning on the basis of principles, there is something suspect about this argument. It suggests that in the current situation—that is, with relatively little demand for luxury primary care—the practice can be endorsed by professional ethics. However, if the demand were great and access were reduced, then the practice would be considered unethical. This means that the definition of ethical practice changes with the situation—in this case, the degree of access to health care. Such situational ethics flies in the face of standard professional principles.

Luxury primary care also undermines cross-subsidized care. For the past 50 years, the American health care system has been dependent on cross-subsidies from patients with good insurance coverage to those with poor coverage or none. For example, a hospital manages to cover the costs of providing care for uninsured patients because it receives payments that exceed the costs of providing care for some well-insured patients. Physicians do the same.

Indeed, such cross-subsidies can be used to justify practices that otherwise might raise serious ethical questions. For instance, some hospitals and doctors solicit wealthy patients from other countries who are willing to pay a premium for care and for deluxe hospital rooms. The key difference between this practice and luxury primary care is presumably that these hospitals and physicians also provide care to the uninsured. Physicians who provide luxury primary care have simply dropped out of the cross-subsidy system, although some have said that they will continue to provide care for some patients who cannot pay the annual fee. This may reduce the damage to a certain extent, but luxury primary care overall will remain a threat to access.

We still might ask whether luxury primary care is more out of line with our professional commitment than are other practices we tolerate. Physicians today choose the communities and the situations in which they are going to practice. Relatively few physicians practice in impoverished inner-city or rural areas; many do not accept patients with Medicaid or those without insurance. As a result, poor people and members of minority racial or ethnic groups generally have less access to health care than other Americans. We have not, as a profession, addressed these issues in a serious fashion. Since we have accepted broad inequities in access to health care in the past, it is difficult to argue that luxury practice should be prohibited.

In this light, the development of luxury primary care might be seen as a crystallizing event. The medical community must be prepared to step forward with ideas and programs that ensure an equitable distribution of health care services. No matter how innovative and attractive luxury primary care is to some patients and physicians, it poses questions about equity. We should identify ways in which luxury primary care can be regulated by the medical profession (perhaps by mandatory cross-subsidies and careful monitoring of the prevalence of such care), while also addressing other threats to access. The questions that luxury primary care poses should remind us that as physicians we have a commitment to the equitable distribution of health care and therefore a duty to address market innovations that could leave some patients without access to care.

Notes

1 Jackson C. Premium practice: when patients pay top dollar for exclusive care. *American Medical News.* September 17, 2001.
2 Belluck P. Doctors' new practices offer deluxe service for deluxe fee. *New York Times.* January 15, 2002:A1.
3 Personal and devoted doctors. *Boston Globe.* January 8, 2002:D8.
4 Moreim EH. *Holding health care accountable: law and the new medical marketplace.* New York: Oxford University Press, 2001.
5 Brennan TA. *Just doctoring: medical ethics in the liberal state.* Berkeley: University of California Press, 1991.
6 Havighurst CC. The changing locus of decision making in the health care sector. *J Health Polit Policy Law* 1986;11:697–735.
7 Sussman AJ, Fairchild DG, Coblyn J, Brennan TA. Primary care compensation at an academic medical center: a model for the mixed-payer environment. *Acad Med* 2001;76: 693–9.
8 Federman AD, Cook EF, Phillips RS, et al. Intention to discontinue care among primary

care patients: the influence of physician behavior and process of care. *J Gen Intern Med* 2001;16:668–74.

9 Fairchild DG, Sussman AJ, Lee TH, Brennan TA. When sick patients switch primary care physicians: the impact on AMCs participating in capitation. *Acad Med* 2000;75:980–5.

10 Mechanic D, McAlpine DD, Rosenthal M. Are patients' office visits with physicians getting shorter? *N Engl J Med* 2001;344:198–204.

11 Mango PD. The case for boutique health care. The McKinsey Quarterly 2002;2:4–6.

12 Haas JS, Cook EF, Puopolo AL, Burstin HR, Cleary PD, Brennan TA. Is the professional satisfaction of general internists associated with patient satisfaction? *J Gen Intern Med* 2000;15:122–8.

13 Gandhi TK, Burstin HR, Cook EF, et al. Drug complications in outpatients. *J Gen Intern Med* 2000;15:149–54.

14 Havighurst CC. *Health care choices: private contracts as instruments of health reform.* Washington, D.C.: AEI Press, 1995.

15 Havighurst C, Blumstein J, Brennan TA. *Health law and policy.* Mineola, N.Y.: Foundation Press, 1999.

16 Colby J, Rice T, Bernstein J, Nelson L. Balance billing under Medicare: protecting beneficiaries and preserving physician participation. *J Health Polit Policy Law* 1995;20:49–74.

17 Massachusetts Medical Society v. Dukakis, 815 F.2d 790 (1st Cir. 1987), cert. denied 484 U.S. 896 (1987).

18 Hall M. A theory of economic informed consent. *Ga L Rev* 1997;31:511–33.

19 Ricks v. Budge, 64 P.2d 208 (Utah 1937).

20 Brennan TA. Ensuring adequate health care for the sick: the challenge of the acquired immunodeficiency syndrome as an occupational disease. *Duke Law J* 1988;1:29–70.

21 Daniels N, Kennedy BP, Kawachi I. Why justice is good for our health: the social determinants of health inequalities. *Daedalus* 1999;128:215–51.

22 Pearson S, Sabin JE, Emanuel EJ. Ethical guidelines for physician compensation based on capitation. *N Engl J Med* 1998;339:689–93.

23 Emanuel EJ. Justice and managed care: four principles for the just allocation of health care resources. *Hastings Cent Rep* 2000;30:8–16.

24 Medical Professionalism Project. Medical professionalism in the new millennium: a physicians' charter. *Lancet* 2002;359:520–2.

Correspondence: Response to "Luxury Primary Care"

To the Editor: The article by Brennan on luxury primary care (April 11 issue)[1] was of particular interest to us as patients of a physician who notified us only two weeks in advance that he would eliminate us from his practice unless we joined MDVIP at a fee of $1,500 per person per year.

Our reaction went from surprise to shock to indignation. For the most part, the services being offered were no different from those we have been receiving—that is, prompt responses to our telephone calls, timely appointments, and adequate examinations and consultation times.

We cannot believe that this kind of medical practice is legal. As Medicare patients, we are entitled to access to our physicians with nothing more than a 20% copayment. Without a doubt, if this practice is allowed to continue, we will have a two-tiered medical system in our country. How sad.

Beverly Sharfstein
Sunny Adler

To the Editor: I have been practicing "luxury" primary care for many years, since I am accessible to all my patients 24 hours a day, 7 days a week, and I do not even charge an annual fee. I allow such access because I strongly believe in practicing patient-centered medicine with joint decision making.

Granted, my practice is small. I am not part of any health maintenance organization, because I do not fit into the mainstream of contemporary medicine. My annual well-woman examination with a pap smear may take

Correspondence: Response to "Luxury Primary Care," from *New England Journal of Medicine*, vol. 347, 618–620. © 2002 by the Massachusetts Medical Society. Reprinted by permission of the publisher.

1. Brennan TA. Luxury primary care—market innovation or threat to access? *N Engl J Med* 2002;346:1165–1168.

up to one and a half hours because I discuss with the patient any health-related concerns she may have. I want my patients to leave my office with all their questions satisfactorily answered and all concerns addressed.

Financially, I am not a huge success. Even as a practicing obstetrician-gynecologist many years ago, my largest gross annual income was less than $200,000. Today, I supplement my income from my office by working elsewhere, and my gross income is about $100,000 per year. But what is money? Serving my patients well is very important to me. Surely, I am not in the minority. I do not want to be in the rat race.

Yasuo Ishida, M.D.

To the Editor: Brennan inadequately addresses the association of many luxury primary care programs with teaching hospitals, where new doctors learn professional ethics and where standards of evidence-based medicine are developed and taught. The general public contributes substantially, through state and federal taxes, to the education and training of new physicians. Should those physicians limit their practices to the wealthiest fraction of our citizenry, when 43 million Americans lack health insurance, our country ranks near the bottom among Western nations in life expectancy and infant mortality, and racial and wealth-based disparities in access to care and outcomes abound?[1] For teaching institutions to promote luxury primary care in the face of these problems is to erode fundamental ethical principles of medicine, such as equity and justice, and such promotion will engender cynicism among trainees and the public.

Martin Donohoe, M.D.

To the Editor: As physicians in the center of the controversy over luxury primary care, we were particularly struck by the absence of the patient's voice in the review by Brennan. The current system of primary care is the creation not of doctors and patients, but of those who pay for care—in general, insurance intermediaries acting on behalf of employers or governments. Since this system is not designed by or for the patients we serve, it is not surprising that there has been widespread dissatisfaction with the results it delivers. When those who pay for services are different from those who receive those services, problems arise. Some patients want something different, and we have responded to that desire.

1. Donohoe MT. Comparing generalist and specialty care: discrepancies, deficiencies, and excesses. *Arch Intern Med* 1998;158:1596–1608.

Our practice is not an answer to the problems of the uninsured, nor is it offered as a solution for all patients or all doctors. Our practice is an answer to the needs of specific persons—patients and doctors—who have felt inadequately served by the system as it exists. We have risked our livelihoods and our reputations in an effort to prove that a better and different way of practicing medicine is possible. We believe that free choice and the marketplace of services and ideas are better alternatives than the status quo. Our success will be measured by our ability to deliver on our promises, as determined by the patients who choose our care.

Steven R. Flier, M.D.

Jordan Busch, M.D.

Nancy H. Corliss, M.D.

To the Editor: Brennan sets out to "examine the . . . ethical issues that arise with [luxury primary care] practices." His chief concern is access, and he concludes with the prescriptive (as opposed to descriptive) statement that "as physicians we have a commitment to the equitable distribution of health care." What is the basis for this statement? Certainly, most people believe that food and shelter are more important than medical care, yet there is no expectation that builders have an obligation to provide for the equitable distribution of housing or that supermarket chains have an obligation to provide for the equitable distribution of food. The origin of Brennan's assertion lies in the concept, beloved by certain policy makers and health economists, of medical exceptionalism. Again, however, beyond the assertion that "medicine is different," there is no argument to sustain such a belief. The distribution of resources belongs in the political arena, and ethical physicians of all stripes can advocate for whatever scheme they are committed to, but clearly equitable distribution is not a problem for the individual physician, no matter how guilty he or she can be made to feel.

Stephen Bohan, M.D.

To the Editor: I take issue with the definition of luxury care given in Brennan's article. "Luxury" is a subjective term that hints at extravagance, exclusivity, and exclusion. It troubles me when this term is used to describe activities that until recently were considered to be quite ordinary— in fact, the standard of care. The half-hour office visit may be a thing of the past, but it seems wrong to regard it as a luxury. In many instances, particularly in the case of an elderly patient with multiple medical problems, more than 15 minutes of a physician's time is a necessity and not a luxury.

I think that the problem that is leading to plans such as "luxury primary care" is the woeful inadequacy of reimbursement for office-based medical care. The current standard for office visits of 15 minutes or less is not a matter of choice, but rather a matter of financial survival. With reimbursement rates as low as they are, a physician has to keep patient turnaround time short in order to keep a practice financially viable. The situation is made worse by the tendency of government to balance its budget at the expense of the medical practitioner. This year, Medicare cut payments to doctors by 5.4%, and additional cuts totaling 17% are anticipated during the next three years.[1] Meanwhile, overhead costs for medical practices continue to climb. For instance, medical-malpractice insurance premiums throughout the country are rising at an average annual rate of 30%.[2] Where will it all lead? Nowhere good, I'm afraid.

Basil K. Lucak, M.D.

To the Editor: I think you should comment on some other losses in the population of physicians who are practicing standard medicine. Could you comment on the ethics of physicians who choose to leave clinical medicine to earn master's degrees in business administration and become physician-executives? Could you comment on physicians who subsequently attend law school and practice law? Could you comment on physicians who retire before becoming enfeebled or incompetent or 65 years of age? Finally, could you comment on the 13th Amendment to the U.S. Constitution and its applicability to persons holding the M.D. degree?

When I attended medical school, the teachers repeatedly articulated the concept that my fellow students and I acquired a special responsibility to society by attending a state-subsidized medical school. In exchange for life-and-death responsibility and hard work, society would offer us respect and remuneration substantially higher than that afforded the average worker.

My perception is that lawyers and bureaucrats have dismantled the implied social contract that was described to me when I was a medical student. Production pressure has diminished "the calling" of being a physician. It comes as no surprise to me that some physicians have found novel ways to support themselves.

James R. Niederlehner, M.D.

1. Pear R. Doctors shunning patients with Medicare. *New York Times.* March 17, 2002:F17.
2. Treaster JB. Doctors face a big jump in insurance. *New York Times.* March 22, 2002:B1.

Dr. Brennan replies:

To the Editor: Bohan and I disagree sharply. I believe that our ethical commitment to patients does create a responsibility to address the distribution of health care resources in the political arena. Medicine is different from other forms of commerce—we adhere to an explicit set of moral principles that give rise to professional responsibilities, including, I believe, the responsibility to address policy issues.

Unlike Flier et al., I do not believe that luxury primary care is a simple matter of choice for patients and doctors. I see it as part of what I believe is a long-term trend toward segmentation of the medical market into the haves and the have-nots. I think that the profession simply cannot tolerate inequalities in the ways in which sick people are treated and must resist libertarian, market-driven changes that create such inequities.

Troyen A. Brennan, M.D.

Limiting Health Care for the Old
Daniel Callahan

In October 1986, Dr. Thomas Starzl of Presbyterian University Hospital in Pittsburgh successfully transplanted a liver into a 76-year-old woman, thereby extending to the elderly patient the most technologically sophisticated and expensive kind of medical treatment available (the typical cost of such an operation is more than $200,000). Not long after that, Congress brought organ transplants under Medicare coverage, thus guaranteeing an even greater range of this form of lifesaving care for older age groups.

That is, on its face, the kind of medical progress we usually hail: a triumph of medical technology and a newfound benefit provided by an established health care program. But at the same time those events were taking place, a government campaign for cost containment was under way, with a special focus on health care to the aged under Medicare. It is not hard to understand why. In 1980 people over age 65—11% of the population—accounted for 29% of the total American health care expenditures of $219.4 billion. By 1986 the elderly accounted for 31% of the total expenditures of $450 billion. Annual Medicare costs are projected to rise from $75 billion in 1986 to $114 billion by the year 2000, and that is in current, not inflated, dollars.

Is it sensible, in the face of the rapidly increasing burden of health care costs for the elderly, to press forward with new and expensive ways of extending their lives? Is it possible even to hope to control costs while simultaneously supporting innovative research, which generates new ways to spend money? Those are now unavoidable questions. Medicare

Daniel Callahan, "Limiting Health Care for the Old?" from *The Nation*, 15 August 1987, 278–282. © 1987 by Daniel Callahan (New York: Simon & Schuster). Reprinted by permission of the publisher.

costs rise at an extraordinary pace, fueled by an increasing number and proportion of the elderly. The fastest growing age group in the United States is comprised of those over age 85, increasing at a rate of about 10% every two years. By the year 2040, it has been projected, the elderly will represent 21% of the population and consume 45% of all health care expenditures. How can costs of that magnitude be borne?

Anyone who works closely with the elderly recognizes that the present Medicare and Medicaid programs are grossly inadequate in meeting their real and full needs. The system fails most notably in providing decent long-term care and medical care that does not constitute a heavy out-of-pocket drain. Members of minority groups and single or widowed women are particularly disadvantaged. How will it be possible, then, to provide the growing number of elderly with even present levels of care, much less to rid the system of its inadequacies and inequities, and at the same time add expensive new technologies?

The straight answer is that it will be impossible to do all those things and, worse still, it may be harmful even to try. It may be so because of the economic burdens that would impose on younger age groups, and because of the requisite skewing of national social priorities too heavily toward health care. But that suggests to both young and old that the key to a happy old age is good health care, which may not be true.

In the past few years three additional concerns about health care for the aged have surfaced. First, an increasingly large share of health care is going to the elderly rather than to youth. The Federal government, for instance, spends six times as much providing health benefits and other social services to those over 65 as it does to those under 18. And, as the demographer Samuel Preston observed in a provocative address to the Population Association of America in 1984, "Transfers from the working-age population to the elderly are also transfers away from children, since the working ages bear far more responsibility for childrearing than do the elderly."

Preston's address had an immediate impact. The mainline senior-citizen advocacy groups accused Preston of fomenting a war between the generations. But the speech also stimulated Minnesota Senator David Durenberger and others to found Americans for Generational Equity (AGE) to promote debate about the burden on future generations, particularly the baby boom cohort, of "our major social insurance programs." Preston's speech and the founding of AGE signaled the outbreak of a struggle over what has come to be called "intergenerational equity," which is now gaining momentum.

The second concern is that the elderly, in dying, consume a disproportionate share of health care costs. "At present," notes Stanford University
economist Victor Fuchs, "the United States spends about 1 percent of the
gross national product on health care for elderly persons who are in their
last year of life. . . . One of the biggest challenges facing policy makers for
the rest of this century will be how to strike an appropriate balance between care for the [elderly] dying and health services for the rest of the
population."

The third issue is summed up in an observation by Dr. Jerome Avorn of
the Harvard Medical School, who wrote in *Daedalus*, "With the exception
of the birth-control pill, [most] of the medical-technology interventions
developed since the 1950s have their most widespread impact on people
who are past their fifties—the further past their fifties, the greater the
impact." Many of the techniques in question were not intended for use on
the elderly. Kidney dialysis, for example, was developed for those between
the ages of 15 and 45. Now some 30% of its recipients are over 65.

The validity of those concerns has been vigorously challenged, as has
the more general assertion that some form of rationing of health care for
the elderly might become necessary. To the charge that old people receive
a disproportionate share of resources, the response has been that assistance to them helps every age group: It relieves the young of the burden of
care they would otherwise have to bear for elderly parents and, since those
young will eventually become old, promises them similar care when they
need it. There is no guarantee, moreover, that any cutback in health care
for the elderly would result in a transfer of the savings directly to the
young. And, some ask, Why should we contemplate restricting care for
the elderly when we wastefully spend hundreds of millions on an inflated
defense budget?

The assertion that too large a share of funds goes to extending the lives
of elderly people who are terminally ill hardly proves that it is an unjust or
unreasonable amount. They are, after all, the most in need. As some important studies have shown, it is exceedingly difficult to know that someone is dying; the most expensive patients, it turns out, are those who were
expected to live but died. That most new technologies benefit the old
more than the young is logical: most of the killer diseases of the young
have now been conquered.

There is little incentive for politicians to think about, much less talk
about, limits on health care for the aged. As John Rother, director of legislation for the American Association of Retired Persons, has observed, "I

think anyone who wasn't a champion of the aged is no longer in Congress." Perhaps also, as Guido Calabresi, dean of the Yale Law School, and his colleague Philip Bobbitt observed in their thoughtful 1978 book *Tragic Choices*, when we are forced to make painful allocation choices, "Evasion, disguise, temporizing . . . [and] averting our eyes enables us to save some lives even when we will not save all."

I believe that we must face this highly troubling issue. Rationing of health care under Medicare is already a fact of life, though rarely labeled as such. The requirement that Medicare recipients pay the first $520 of hospital care costs, the cutoff of reimbursement for care after 60 days, and the failure to cover long-term care are nothing other than allocation and cost-saving devices. As sensitive as it is to the senior citizen vote, the Reagan Administration agreed only grudgingly to support catastrophic health care coverage for the elderly (a benefit that will not help very many of them), and it has already expressed its opposition to the recently passed House version of the bill. It is bound to be far more resistant to long-term health care coverage, as will any administration.

But there are reasons other than the economics to think about health care for the elderly. The coming economic crisis provides a much needed opportunity to ask some deeper questions. Just what is it that we want medicine to do for us as we age? Other cultures have believed that aging should be accepted, and that it should be in part a time of preparation for death. Our culture seems increasingly to dispute that view, preferring instead, it often seems, to think of aging as hardly more than another disease, to be fought and rejected. Which view is correct?

Let me interject my own opinion. The future goal of medical science should be to improve the quality of old people's lives, not to lengthen them. In its long-standing ambition to forestall death, medicine has reached its last frontier in the care of the aged. Of course children and young adults still die of maladies that are open to potential cure; but the highest proportion of the dying (70%) are over 65. If death is ever to be humbled, that is where endless work remains to be done. But however tempting the challenge of that last frontier, medicine should restrain itself. To do otherwise would mean neglecting the needs of other age groups and of the old themselves.

Our culture has worked hard to redefine old age as a time of liberation, not decline, a time of travel, of new ventures in education and self-discovery, of the ever accessible tennis court or golf course and of delightfully periodic but thankfully brief visits from well-behaved grandchildren.

That is, to be sure, an idealized picture, but it arouses hopes that spur medicine to wage an aggressive war against the infirmities of old age. As we have seen, the costs of such a war would be prohibitive. No matter how much is spent the ultimate problem will still remain: people will grow old and die. Worse still, by pretending that old age can be turned into a kind of endless middle age, we rob it of meaning and significance for the elderly.

There is a plausible alternative: a fresh vision of what it means to live a decently long and adequate life, what might be called a "natural life span." Earlier generations accepted the idea that there was a natural life span— the biblical norm of three score and ten captures that notion (even though in fact that was a much longer life span than was typical in ancient times). It is an idea well worth reconsidering and would provide us with a meaningful and realizable goal. Modern medicine and biology have done much, however, to wean us from that kind of thinking. They have insinuated the belief that the average life span is not a natural fact at all, but instead one that is strictly dependent on the state of medical knowledge and skill. And there is much to that belief as a statistical fact: The average life expectancy continues to increase, with no end in sight.

But that is not what I think we ought to mean by a natural life span. We need a notion of a full life that is based on some deeper understanding of human needs and possibilities, not on the state of medical technology or its potential. We should think of a natural life span as the achievement of a life that is sufficiently long to take advantage of those opportunities life typically offers and that we ordinarily regard as its prime benefits—loving and "living," raising a family, engaging in work that is satisfying, reading, thinking, cherishing our friends and families. People differ on what might be a full natural life span; my view is that it can be achieved by the late 70s or early 80s.

A longer life does not guarantee a better life. No matter how long medicine enables people to live, death at any time—at age 90 or 100 or 110— would frustrate some possibility, some as-yet-unrealized goal. The easily preventable death of a young child is an outrage. Death from an incurable disease of someone in the prime of young adulthood is a tragedy. But death at an old age, after a long and full life, is simply sad, a part of life itself.

As it confronts aging, medicine should have as its specific goals the averting of premature death, that is, death prior to the completion of a natural life span, and thereafter, the relief of suffering. It should pursue those goals so that the elderly can finish out their years with as little needless pain as possible—and with as much vitality as can be generated in contributing to the welfare of younger age groups and to the community of which they are a part. Above all, the elderly need to have a sense of the meaning and significance of their stage in life, one that is not dependent on economic productivity or physical vigor.

What would medicine oriented toward the relief of suffering rather than the deliberate extension of life be like? We do not have a clear answer to that question, so long-standing, central, and persistent has been medicine's preoccupation with the struggle against death. But the hospice movement is providing us with much guidance. It has learned how to distinguish between the relief of suffering and the lengthening of life. Greater control by elderly persons over their own dying—and particularly an enforceable right to refuse aggressive life-extending treatment—is a minimal goal.

What does this have to do with the rising cost of health care for the elderly? Everything. The indefinite extension of life combined with an insatiable ambition to improve the health of the elderly is a recipe for monomania and bottomless spending. It fails to put health in its proper place as only one among many human goods. It fails to accept aging and death as part of the human condition. It fails to present to younger generations a model of wise stewardship.

How might we devise a plan to limit the costs of health care for the aged under public entitlement programs that is fair, humane and sensitive to their special requirements and dignity? Let me suggest three principles to undergird a quest for limits. First, government has a duty, based on our collective social obligations, to help people live out a natural life span but not to help medically extend life beyond that point. Second, government is obliged to develop under its research subsidies, and to pay for under its entitlement programs, only the kind and degree of life-extending technology necessary for medicine to achieve and serve the aim of a natural life span. Third, beyond the point of a natural life span, government should provide only the means necessary for the relief of suffering, not those for life-extending technology.

A system based on those principles would not immediately bring down the cost of care of the elderly; it would add cost. But it would set in place the beginning of a new understanding of old age, one that would admit of eventual stabilization and limits. The elderly will not be served by a belief that only a lack of resources, better financing mechanisms, or political power stands between them and the limitations of their bodies. The good of younger age groups will not be served by inspiring in them a desire to live to an old age that maintains the vitality of youth indefinitely, as if old age were nothing but a sign that medicine has failed in its mission. The future of our society will not be served by allowing expenditures on health care for the elderly to escalate endlessly and uncontrollably, fueled by the false altruistic belief that anything less is to deny the elderly their dignity. Nor will it be aided by the pervasive kind of self-serving argument that urges the young to support such a crusade because they will eventually benefit from it also.

We require instead an understanding of the process of aging and death that looks to our obligation to the young and to the future, that recognizes the necessity of limits and the acceptance of decline and death, and that values the old for their age and not for their continuing youthful vitality. In the name of accepting the elderly and repudiating discrimination against them, we have succeeded mainly in pretending that, with enough will and money, the unpleasant part of old age can be abolished. In the name of medical progress we have carried out a relentless war against death and decline, failing to ask in any probing way if that will give us a better society for all.

Scapegoating the Aged: Intergenerational Equity and Age-Based Rationing

Robert H. Binstock

The Public Policy Context: Compassionate Ageism and the "Old-Age Welfare State"

From the Social Security Act of 1935 through 1970s, American policies toward older persons have been adopted and amended in substantially different social, economic, and political contexts. Interpretations of the original goals of such policies vary widely (Achenbaum 1983; Campion 1984; Cohen 1985b; David 1985; Derthick 1979; Graebner 1980; Harris 1966; Holtzman 1963; Marmor 1970).

Regardless of the original intent of various policies toward aging, by the late 1960s and early 1970s a common theme was taking shape: Through the cumulative impact of many disparate legislative actions, American society had adopted and financed a number of age-categorical benefit programs and tax and price subsidies for which eligibility is not determined by need. Through Social Security, Medicare, the Older Americans Act, and a variety of other measures, older persons were exempted from the screenings that are customarily applied to other Americans in order to determine whether they are worthy of public help.

This theme was strengthened as a number of old-age-based interest groups articulated compassionate stereotypes of older persons (Binstock 1972; Pratt 1976). These advocates for the aged told us repeatedly that the elderly are poor, frail, socially dependent, objects of discrimination, and, above all, *deserving* (Kalish 1979).

Through this compassionate ageism—the attribution of the same characteristics, status, and just deserts to the elderly—advocates managed

Robert H. Binstock, "The Oldest Old and Intergenerational Equity," in *The Oldest Old*, Richard M. Suzman, David P. Wells, and Kenneth G. Manton, eds., pp. 394–417 (New York: Oxford University Press, 1992).

to artificially homogenize, package, label, and market a heterogeneous group of older persons as "the aged" (Binstock 1983). However, ageism, in contrast with racism, has provided many benefits to older persons (Kutza 1981).

Because older persons came to be stereotyped as the "deserving poor," programs for the aged have not been subject to the disdain and stigmatization attached to other welfare programs in American political culture. In truth, of course, any of the "deserving" needs for collective assistance that have been symbolized by compassionate old-age stereotypes can be found among persons of all ages. Yet, the great bulk of our social-welfare and health expenditures is for benefits to the aged.

The Emergence of the Aged as Scapegoat

Since 1978, however, the long-standing compassionate stereotypes of older persons have been undergoing an extraordinary reversal (Binstock 1983). Older persons have come to be portrayed as one of the more flourishing and powerful groups in American society and have been attacked as a burdensome responsibility. These new stereotypes, devoid of compassion, are

1. The aged are relatively well off—not poor, but in great economic shape.

2. The aged are a potent political force because there are so many of them and they all vote in their self-interest; this "senior power" explains why more than one-quarter of the annual federal budget is spent on benefits to the aged.

3. Because of demographic changes, the aged are becoming more numerous and politically powerful, and will claim even more benefits and substantially larger proportions of the federal budget. They are already costing too much, and in the future will pose an unsustainable burden for the American economy.

Even as the earlier compassionate stereotypes of older persons were partially unwarranted, so are these current stereotypes. They are generated by applying simplistic assumptions and aggregate statistics to a group called "the aged" in order to gloss over complexities. If one chooses to compare changes in the median or average income of all older persons with changes in the income of other groups, one can conclude that the aged are relatively well off and ignore millions of older persons who are in dire economic circumstances (Smeeding 1990). If one wishes to ignore abundant evidence to the contrary (Hudson and Strate 1985; Jacobs 1990), one can assume that the votes of older persons are determined by issues, and one particular issue above all others, which they will respond to with self-interest, and that their self-interests will be common. If one pretends that outlays for Medicare, Old Age Insurance, and other policies are mechanistically determined by demographics rather than by legislative and administrative decisions, one can conclude that benefits to the aged constitute an unsustainable burden for the American economy. But extrapolation from existing policies and institutional arrangements is a poor mode of prediction.

The new stereotypes of older persons began to appear in the late 1970s. One element in the change was a tremendous growth in the amount of federal funds expended on benefits to the aging, which journalists (Samuelson 1978) and academicians (Hudson 1978) began to notice and publicize in the late 1970s. By 1982 an economist in the U.S. Office of Management and Budget (Torrey 1982) had reframed the classical tradeoff metaphor of political economy from "guns versus butter" to "guns versus canes." By the late 1980s, the proportion of the annual federal budget being spent on benefits to the aging had remained at about 26% for more than a decade (U.S. Senate 1988) and had been widely recognized as one of the few large expenditure categories in the federal budget (along with national defense and interest on the national debt).

Another element in the reversal of old-age stereotypes was dramatic improvement in the aggregate status of older Americans, in large measure due to the impact of federal benefit programs.

Regardless of specific causes, the reversal of stereotypes continued throughout the 1980s to the point where the new stereotypes can now be readily observed in popular culture. Typical of contemporary depictions of older persons was a cover story in *Time Magazine* entitled "Grays on the Go" (Gibbs 1988). It was filled with pictures of senior surfers, swingers, and softball players. Older persons were pictured as America's new elite—healthy, wealthy, powerful, and "staging history's biggest retirement party."

A dominant theme in such portrayals of older persons is that their selfishness is ruining the nation. The *New Republic* highlighted this motif early in 1988 with a cover displaying "Greedy Geezers." Or, as a *New York Times* Op-Ed article was headlined: "Elderly, Affluent—and Selfish" (Longman 1989).

In serious forums of public discourse these new stereotypes have bolstered the use of the aged as a scapegoat for an impressive list of American problems. As social psychologist Gordon Allport observed in his classic work on the *ABC's of Scapegoating:* "An issue seems nicely simplified if we blame a group or class of people rather than the complex course of social and historical forces" (1959, 13–14).

Advocates for children and demographer Samuel Preston (1984) have blamed the political power of the elderly for the plight of youngsters who have inadequate nutrition, health care, and education and lack supportive family environments. Former secretary of commerce Peter Peterson (1987) has suggested that a prerequisite for the United States to regain its stature as a first-class power in the world economy is a sharp reduction in programs benefiting older Americans.

Perhaps the most serious scapegoating of the aged—in terms of the vulnerability of older persons, the oldest old, and, maybe, of all persons in our society—has been in the area of health care. A widespread concern about high rates of inflation in health care costs has been refocused in the past few years from health care providers, suppliers, administrators, and insurers—the parties that are responsible for setting the prices of care—to the elderly patients for whom health care is provided and who pay for more than 40% of their aggregate care (U.S. House of Representatives 1989, 8).

Americans aged 65 and older, about 12% of our population, account for one-third of the nation's annual health-care expenditures (U.S. House of Representatives 1989, 4). Because the elderly population is growing, absolutely and proportionately, health care costs for older persons have been depicted as an unsustainable burden, or as ethicist Daniel Callahan has put it, "a great fiscal black hole" that will absorb an unlimited amount of our national resources (1987, 17). Indeed, because of concerns for health care costs of the old, in 1984 the then Governor of Colorado, Richard Lamm, was widely reported to have pronounced that terminally ill old people have a "duty to die and get out of the way" (Slater 1984).

Intergenerational Equity: Justice between Age Groups

"Justice between age groups" (Daniels 1983) has become a metaphor for concerns that ever increasing health care costs in the United States will bring about far more rationing of acute health care than we have thus far experienced informally (Blank 1988).

There is no inherent reason, of course, why issues of justice in allocating health care resources need to be framed on the basis of age. One can frame tradeoffs just as easily within age groups or without regard to age. In fact, health care resources—like most other goods and services in the United States—have long been allocated on the basis of social class and ability to pay (Churchill 1987). Many procedures—even relatively low-cost ones, such as immunization—are not readily available to persons of low economic and social status (Hiatt 1987).

Nonetheless, old age came sharply into focus as a prime target for stepped-up acute care rationing in the past decade. In a 1983 speech, economist Alan Greenspan, now chairman of the Federal Reserve Board, stated that 30% of Medicare is annually expended on 5 to 6% of Medicare eligibles who die within the year. He pointedly considered whether it is worth it. (Schulte 1983). Richard Lamm says that he was misquoted in 1984 when he was reported as urging older persons to die in order to make room for the young (Slater 1984), but he has been delivering the same message repeatedly since then, in only somewhat more delicately worded fashion (e.g., Lamm 1987, 1989a).

During the last half of the 1980s, this focus spread to a number of forums. Philosophers generated principles of equity to undergird "justice between age groups" in the provision of health care (e.g., Daniels 1988), rather than, for instance, justice between rich and poor. Conferences and books explicitly addressed the issue of "Should Health Care Be Rationed by Age?" (e.g., Smeeding et al. 1987), and biomedical ethicists turned to examining the economics of terminal illness (Veatch 1988) and "assisted suicide" in old age (Battin 1987).

In the context of this ongoing dialogue on old-age-based health care rationing, the swiftly increasing oldest-old population may well develop as the leading symbol for "runaway" health costs. Persons aged 85 and older, for instance, stand out—even among elderly persons—as high users of health-care resources.

The greater numbers of persons who will be in the oldest-old category, combined with their current high rates of health care use, lead to projections that Medicare costs for the oldest old may increase sixfold by the year 2040, as estimated in constant, inflation-adjusted dollars (Schneider and Guralnik 1990).

Even in the mid-1980s, as issues of health care costs and allocations began to be framed as tradeoffs between age groups, it did "not take much imagination to envision that a stereotyped group termed the 'oldest old' will be assembled in the front row of the trading block" (Binstock 1985,

433). And indeed, they have been by ethicist Daniel Callahan, who is willing to transcend the bounds of traditional Judeo-Christian morality (Post 1991) regarding the sanctity of human life.

In a book entitled *Setting Limits: Medical Goals in an Aging Society*, Callahan proposes that life-saving health care should be officially forbidden to all American citizens who are of an advanced age category. He depicts the elderly as "a new social threat" and a "demographic, economic, and medical avalanche . . . that could ultimately (and perhaps already) do great harm" (1987, 20). Callahan's remedy for this threat is to use "age as a specific criterion for the allocation and limitation of health care" (23), by denying life-extending health care—as a matter of public policy—to persons who are aged in their "late 70s or early 80s" and/or have 'lived out a natural life span' " (171).

Although Callahan's arguments are seriously flawed (Binstock and Kahana 1988), his proposal received a great deal of national attention. It was reviewed in national magazines, the *New York Times*, the *Washington Post*, the *Wall Street Journal*, and almost every relevant professional and scholarly journal and newsletter. Callahan himself was and continues to be invited to present and/or debate his proposal in a number of public forums throughout the country, and he has reiterated his viewpoint in a recent book (Callahan 1990). It appears that his proposal to forbid life-saving care to the oldest among us has come to be rather firmly embedded in public discourse concerning health care policies in the United States.

Such proposals are likely to persist, albeit with refinements. And they will probably stay focused on very old persons because of preoccupations with financing and outlays for the Medicare program, the biggest single source of payment for health care in America (Health Care Financing Administration 1987). Moreover, Medicare, widely perceived as the "health program for the elderly," is a prime target for cost containment reforms because its approaches to paying for care affect the financial incentives of a very high percentage of American hospitals, nursing homes, physicians, and other health care providers and suppliers.

Increasing Dependency Ratios

"Increasing dependency ratios," conventionally expressed as the size of the retired population relative to the working population, has become a metaphor for anxieties about the economic burdens of population aging. This construct grossly distorts the issues involved because it is largely an artifact of an existing policy, Social Security, that finances benefits to retirees through a tax based on the paychecks of workers. It does not capture the range of major elements that determine whether a society is economically capable of supporting dependents within it.

The most fundamental problem with this construct lies in using the number or proportion of workers in a society in order to assess the productive capacity of the economy. Productive capacity is a function of a variety of factors—including capital, natural resources, balance of trade, and technological innovation—as well as number of workers. Hence, issues involving productive capacity and number of workers should be expressed in terms of "productivity per worker" in order to take account of an appropriately full range of macroeconomic variables (Committee on an Aging Society 1986; Habib 1990).

More specific flaws in common usage of dependency ratios express the ubiquitous impact of ageism in the framing of issues. Age categories are used to estimate the numbers of workers and retirees—rather than actual and projected labor force participation rates—even though the two approaches can yield substantially different results. In addition, the focus on retirees as the "dependent population" ignores the fact that many retired older persons are economically independent. It also ignores children and unemployed adults of any age who are economically dependent; for instance, research has indicated that a decline in "youth dependency" during the decades ahead may well moderate or even dominate the economic significance of projected increases in "elderly dependency" (Crown 1985; Habib 1990).

Nevertheless, discussions of increasing dependency ratios have generated several assumptions that may be unwarranted: First, we will need a far greater number of workers in the decades ahead than is projected from current age norms for entering and retiring from the labor force. Second, older persons who retire in the context of contemporary policies, many of whom engage in unpaid productive activities (Committee on an Aging Society 1986), will want to and be able to work for pay in the future if incentives to retire and the ages associated with them are marginally adjusted. Third, it is assumed that there will be employer demand for such workers.

The Political Power of the Aged

"The political power of the aged" is still another metaphor frequently used to misframe issues in terms of age group conflicts (e.g., Chakravarty and Weisman 1988). Although older persons have constituted 16.7 to 21% of those who voted in national elections during the 1980s (U.S. Senate 1988, 11), election exit polls have demonstrated repeatedly that the votes of older persons are distributed among candidates in about the same proportions as the votes of other age groups of citizens (*New York Times*/CBS News Poll 1980, 1982, 1984, 1986, 1988). Even in the context of a state or local referendum that presents a specific issue, rather than candidates, for balloting—such as propositions to cap local property taxes or to finance public schools—old age is not a statistically significant variable associated with the distribution of votes (Chomitz 1987).

These data should not be surprising because there is no sound reason to expect that a cohort of persons would suddenly become homogenized in self-interests and political behavior when it reaches the old-age category (Simon 1985). Diversity among older persons may be at least as great with respect to political attitudes and behavior as it is in relation to economic, social, and other characteristics (Hudson and Strate 1985).

Moreover, the scholarly literature indicates that organized demands of older persons have had little to do with the enactment and amendment of the major old-age policies such as Social Security and Medicare. Rather, such actions have been largely attributable to the initiatives of public officials in the White House, Congress, and the bureaucracy who have focused on their own agendas for social and economic policy (Cohen 1985a; Derthick 1979; Hudson and Strate 1985; Jacobs 1990; Light 1985).

At present, the old age interest organizations seem to be functioning as what political scientist Heclo (1984) terms an "anti-redistributive veto force" in American politics. Even in this so-called veto role, however, the force of old age interests appears to be relatively weak.

A number of public policy decisions that are conventionally perceived as adverse to the self-interests of older persons proved to be politically feasible in the 1980s through changes in Medicare, Social Security, and other programs. Medicare deductibles, copayments, and Part B premiums have increased continuously. Old Age Insurance (OAI) benefits have become subject to taxation. The legislated formula for cost-of-living-adjustments (COLAS) to OAI benefits has been rendered less generous. Most recently, the politics of enacting and repealing of the Catastrophic Coverage Act clearly illustrated that older persons are not a homogeneous group, either politically or in terms of self-interests.

Despite these facts, the image of so-called senior power persists because it serves certain purposes. It is used by journalists as a tabloid symbol to simplify the complexities of politics. It is marketed by the leaders of old age–based organizations who have many incentives to inflate the size of the constituency for which they speak, even if they need to homogenize it artificially in order to do so. It is attacked by those who would like to see greater resources allocated to their causes and who depict the selfishness of the aged as the root of many problems (Longman 1987).

Transcending Intergenerational Equity: Perspectives on Old Age–Based Health Care Rationing

These examples of current metaphors in the politics of health and social welfare allocations may be sufficient to illustrate that issues are being framed in terms of conflicts between age groups; that these issues are frequently constructed from spurious and unwarranted assumptions; and that the emergence of the oldest old within these scenarios tends to exacerbate the implications of the issues that have been framed.

The lesson to be drawn from this is *not* that research on the oldest old should cease or be muted. Indeed, multidimensional knowledge about persons who are in their late 80s and older will be essential for coping with the challenges posed by population aging. It is important to note, however, that the issues of intergenerational equity—although arbitrary and flawed—have focused the social policy agenda and diverted attention from other ways of viewing tradeoffs and options available to us that may be more accurate and propitious.

The lesson *is* that any description of the axis upon which equity is to be judged tends to circumscribe the major options available for rendering justice. If we can perceive issues that express equity in ways other than intergenerational tradeoffs (Heclo 1988; Kingson, Hirshorn, and Cornman 1986; Neugarten and Neugarten 1986; Wisensale 1988), those alternative issues may generate a series of new practical choices for public and private institutional arrangements in the decades ahead. It is not within the scope of this discussion to set forth a blueprint for such arrangements. But it is feasible to illustrate the principle by briefly considering some of the ways in which issues of health resources allocation, presently expressed in terms of old age–based rationing proposals, can be viewed in other terms.

Many contemporary discussions about old age–based rationing are laden with misperceptions of what is actually happening in the world of health care for elderly Americans. Physicians are viewed as blindly pursuing a "heroic model" of medicine (see Cassel and Neugarten 1991) in which no cost or form of intervention will be spared in attempting to extend the lives of persons who are already near the end of their natural life course. These expenditures and interventions are seen as largely futile and wasteful, especially when applied to the very old. And their elimination, through one means or another, is perceived as an important measure for reducing health care costs, particularly because of the swiftly increasing size of the oldest-old population.

But the decision processes through which physicians actually decide whether and how to treat elderly patients are not widely known. The benefits such patients receive from treatments are not understood, either in comparison with younger patients or in terms of cost effectiveness for society. Frequently quoted statistics concerning health care costs are often unexamined with respect to their significance.

The Myth of Overly Aggressive, High-Technology Care for the Elderly

A central theme in most current discussions of whether American society should deny or limit health care to older persons is that costly, high-technology medicine is used too frequently and wastefully in treating elderly patients (e.g., Callahan 1987; Daniels 1988; U.S. Congress 1987). For some years the press has provided dramatic accounts of organ transplants and other forms of surgery on persons in their 70s, 80s, and 90s (e.g., Koenig 1986), as well as reports of legal issues involving the extended ordeals of older patients who linger on the edge of death in hospitals, sustained only by mechanical breathing ventilators or nutrition obtained intravenously or through tube feeding (e.g., Kleiman 1985).

However, the popular conception that elderly persons are frequently subject to "Faustian technologies" of intensive care (Lamm 1989a, 6) against their wishes is wrong (Schwartz and Reilly 1986). The majority of the funds expended on health care for the aged in the United States are not for dramatic technological interventions or even for hospitals. In 1988 nursing homes accounted for 21% of health expenditures on older persons, yet only a negligible proportion of elderly nursing-home patients receive life-sustaining technologies (U.S. Congress 1987, 12). A wide range of nonhospital and nonphysician health services—such as prescription drugs, dental care, home health care, vision and hearing aids, and medical equipment and supplies—totaled 16% of expenditures, and outpatient and inpatient physician fees were 22%. The remaining 41% was for payments to hospitals (U.S. House of Representatives 1989, 21).

Studies in both the United States (Scitovsky 1984) and Canada (Roos, Montgomery, and Roos 1987) indicate that aggressive acute care medical interventions are comparable across adult age groups in the last years of life, although elderly persons are far more likely to incur expenses for nursing homes and home care services. In fact, a study of several hundred older persons who died within a 12-month period indicates that severely impaired geriatric patients who received only supportive care—and little of it from hospitals and physicians—averaged only slightly fewer expenses for the year (amounting to about 8% less) than the most expensive decedents, who were treated aggressively with high-technology measures (Scitovsky 1988).

Old age, as a single factor or independent variable, is a poor predictor of whether a medical intervention will be "wasted," even for highly technical and aggressive medical interventions (see Jahnigen and Binstock 1991). Moreover, experience with advanced medical technologies—such as those used in renal dialysis, liver transplantation, and heart transplantation—shows that those older patients who are selected for such procedures unquestionably benefit from them, sometimes more than younger patients (Evans 1991). In certain cases, even transplantations are the most cost-effective mode of treatment. For example, kidney transplant recipients whose new organs function satisfactorily incur far lower treatment expenses than dialysis patients (Evans et al. 1987; Evans, Manninen, and Thompson 1989).

At the same time, the caricature of contemporary physicians as Don Quixotes who will tilt at "death as an enemy," regardless of cost and prognosis, misses the mark badly. Transplantation specialists, for example, take great care to select older candidates for surgery who have outstanding prospects for survival and benefit (Evans 1991). Furthermore, it is clear that physicians generally recognize the futility of many interventions for older persons, depending on disease and level of function (Gillick 1988; La Puma et al. 1988; Miles and Ryder 1985; Scitovsky 1988; Youngner et al. 1985).

Even if health care treatment of older persons is not wasteful or overly aggressive, it is not always successful. Alan Greenspan's 1983 pronouncement (Schulte 1983) that a high proportion of Medicare expenditures is accounted for by a small proportion of Medicare enrollees who die within the year was basically correct. About 6% of Medicare enrollees who die within a year account for about 28% of Medicare's annual expenditures (Lubitz and Prihoda 1984). In 1987, when the total Medicare expenditure was $81 billion (Letsch, Levit, and Waldo 1988), this would mean that about $22.6 billion in Medicare funds was used to reimburse health care for about 6% of Medicare eligibles who died.

Suppose it were possible, both clinically and ethically, to identify prospectively those Medicare patients who were going to die within the year, and whose treatment would be *comparatively costly*, to choose not to undertake aggressive treatment of them, and thereby to save unnecessary health care costs? How much would be saved in terms of Medicare resources and the nation's annual health expenditures? To the extent that it is possible to estimate, not very much.

The best available nationwide study (Lubitz and Prihoda 1984) found that in 1978 only 3% of Medicare-eligible decedents had reimbursements of $20,000 or more, and they accounted for 3.5% of total Medicare expenditures that year. This $20,000 or more per capita figure for the high cost of Medicare decedents would undoubtedly be much larger today because health care costs have increased substantially in the ensuing years (U.S. House of Representatives 1989, 10).

Placing these findings in the context of a more recent year, the 3.5% of Medicare spent on high-cost decedents in 1978 would have yielded a total of $2.84 billion for 1987. To be sure, changing medical practices such as the introduction of high-cost technologies and low-cost hospice programs may have had the net effect of increasing or decreasing the percentage of Medicare spent on high-cost decedents since 1978. Even an increase of 1 or 2%, however, would not substantially change the general picture.

In the context of 1987, when national health care expenditures were over $500 billion and Medicare expenditures were $81 billion, saving an estimated $2.84 billion seems negligible. If there is some sort of health care cost crisis in the United States, saving such an amount in itself would hardly make a dent in the overall situation.

Even if our nation were firmly resolved, as a matter of public policy, to eliminate all wasteful and unnecessary health care expenditures, and even if it was ethically palatable to do so, would it be possible to eliminate such "waste" by not treating Medicare patients who are likely to be expensive decedents? Only, apparently, if we are willing not to treat costly patients who will recover—to throw away those high-cost patients who would survive into the same "wastebasket" as costly decedents. The study by Lubitz and Prihoda (1984) found about the same numbers of survivors and decedents in the high-cost patient category and about the same amount of aggregate expenditures on them. Of 49,000 Medicare enrollees in the high-cost category, 25,000 survived and 24,000 died.

Conclusion

This discussion of perspectives on old age–based health care rationing represents but one example of how contemporary dilemmas can be perceived in terms that express neither compassionate and dispassionate ageism nor conflicts between age groups. Whether such perceptions are more accurate or even more propitious ways to frame issues is certainly open to debate. They have been offered to illustrate that preoccupations with stereotypes, conventional wisdom, and existing policies and institutional arrangements can divert us from seeking alternative ways to anticipate and deal with the implications of population aging and other societal challenges.

Even as we generate valuable knowledge about the oldest-old population to inform our choices for the future, it is especially important that we examine the principles of equity implicit in the choices that we frame. If we allow our thinking to be confined by an agenda of intergenerational equity issues, and by our current policies and the principles that they have come to reflect, we may very well find ourselves engaged in policy debates on issues of age-group conflict that are far worse than those we have experienced to date: trading off the value of one human life against another as a matter of official policy.

Ultimately, the principles of equity that we use to describe our choices will be far more important than data and policy analyses for shaping the quality of life and the nature of justice in our society, and for the oldest old among us.

Note

The original article has been abridged for this edition.

References

Achenbaum, W.A. 1983. *Shades of Gray: Old Age, American Values, and Federal Policies since 1920*. Boston: Little, Brown.

Allport, G.W. 1959. *ABC's of Scapegoating*. New York: Anti-Defamation League of B'nai B'rith.

Battin, M.P. 1987. Choosing the Time to Die: The Ethics and Economics of Suicide in Old Age. In *Ethical Dimensions of Geriatric Care*, ed. S. Spicker, 161–189. Dordrect, Holland: Reidel.

Binstock, R.H. 1972. Interest-group Liberalism and the Politics of Aging. *The Gerontologist* 12:265–80.

——. 1983. The Aged as Scapegoat. *The Gerontologist* 23:136–43.

——. 1985. The Oldest-Old: A Fresh Perspective or Compassionate Ageism Revisited? *Milbank Memorial Fund Quarterly/Health and Society* 63:420–51.

Binstock, R.H., and J. Kahana. 1988. An Essay on *Setting Limits: Medical Goals in an Aging Society*, by D. Callahan. *The Gerontologist* 28:424–26.

Blank, R.H. 1988. *Rationing Medicine*. New York: Columbia University Press.

Callahan, D. 1987. *Setting Limits: Medical Goals in an Aging Society*. New York: Simon and Schuster.

——. 1990. *What Kind of Life: The Limits of Medical Progress*. New York: Simon and Schuster.

Campion, F.D. 1984. *The AMA and U.S. Health Policy since 1940*. Chicago: Chicago Review Press.

Cassel, C.K., and B.L. Neugarten. 1991. The Goals of Medicine in an Aging Society. In *Too Old for Health Care?: Controversies in Medicine, Law, Economics, and Ethics*, eds. R.H. Binstock and S.G. Post, 75–91. Baltimore, Md.: Johns Hopkins University Press.

Chakravarty, S.N., and K. Weisman. 1988. Consuming Our Children? *Forbes* 142:222–32.

Chomitz, K.M. 1987. Demographic Influences on Local Public Education Expenditures: A Review of Econometric Evidence. In *Demographic Change and the Well-Being of Children and the Elderly*, eds. Committee on Population, Commission on Behavioral and Social Sciences Education, National Research Council, 45–53. Washington: National Academy Press.

Churchill, L.R. 1987. *Rationing Health Care in America: Perceptions and Principles of Justice*. Notre Dame, Ind.: University of Notre Dame Press.

Clark, R.L. 1990. Income Maintenance Policies in the United States. In *Handbook of Aging and the Social Sciences*, 3rd ed., eds. R.H. Binstock and L.K. George, 382–97. San Diego, Calif.: Academic Press.

Cohen, W.J. 1985a. Securing Social Security. *New Leader* 66:5–8.

——. 1985b. Reflections on the Enactment of Medicare and Medicaid. *Health Care Financing Review* (Annual Supplement):3–11.

Committee on an Aging Society, Institute of Medicine and National Research Council. 1986. *America's Aging: Productive Roles in an Older Society*. Washington: National Academy Press.

Crown, W. 1985. Some Thoughts on Reformulating the Dependency Ratio. *The Gerontologist* 25:166–71.

Daniels, N. 1983. Justice between Age Groups: Am I My Parents' Keeper? *Milbank Memorial Fund Quarterly/Health and Society* 61(3):489–522.

———. 1988. *Am I My Parents' Keeper? An Essay on Justice between the Young and the Old.* New York: Oxford University Press.

David, S.I. 1985. *With Dignity, the Search for Medicare and Medicaid.* Westport, Conn.: Greenwood Press.

Derthick, M. 1979. *Policymaking for Social Security.* Washington: Brookings Institution.

Evans, R.W. 1991. Advanced Medical Technology and Elderly People. In *Too Old for Health Care? Controversies in Medicine, Law, Economics, and Ethics,* eds. R.H. Binstock and S.G. Post, 44–74. Baltimore, Md.: Johns Hopkins University Press.

Evans, R.W., D.L. Manninen, L.P. Garrison, Jr., and L.G. Hart. 1987. *Special Report: Findings from the National Kidney Dialysis and Kidney Transplantation Study.* Baltimore, Md.: Health Care Financing Administration (HCFA pub. no. 03230).

Evans, R.W., D.L. Manninen, and C. Thompson. 1989. *A Cost and Outcome Analysis of Kidney Transplantation: The Implications of Initial Immunosuppressive Protocol and Diabetes.* Seattle, Wash.: Battelle Human Affairs Research Centers.

Gibbs, N.R. 1988. Grays on the Go. *Time,* 131(8):66–75.

Gillick, M. 1988. Limiting Medical Care: Physicians' Beliefs, Physicians' Behavior. *Journal of the American Geriatric Society* 36:747–52.

Graebner, W. 1980. *A History of Retirement: The Meanings and Functions of an American Institution, 1885–1978.* New Haven, Conn.: Yale University Press.

Habib, J. 1990. The Economy and the Aged. In *Handbook of Aging and the Social Sciences,* 3rd ed., eds. R.H. Binstock and L.K. George, 328–45. San Diego, Calif.: Academic Press.

Harris, R. 1966. *A Sacred Trust.* New York: American Library.

Health Care Financing Administration. 1987. National Health Expenditures, 1986–2000. *Health Care Financing Review* 8(4):1–36.

Heclo, H. 1984. The Political Foundations of Anti-Poverty Policy. Paper prepared for the IRP conference, *Poverty and Policy: Retrospect and Prospects,* 6–8. Madison, Wis.: Institute for Research on Poverty.

———. 1988. Generational Politics. In *The Vulnerable,* eds. J.L. Palmer, T. Smeeding, and B.B. Torrey, 381–411. Washington: Urban Institute Press.

Hiatt, H.H. 1987. *America's Health in the Balance: Choice or Change?* New York: Harper and Row.

Holtzman, A. 1963. *The Townsend Movement: A Political Study.* New York: Bookman.

Hudson, R.B. 1978. The "Graying" of the Federal Budget and Its Consequences for Old Age Policy. *The Gerontologist* 18:428–40.

Hudson, R.B., and J. Strate. 1985. Aging and Political Systems. In *Handbook of Aging and the Social Sciences,* 2nd ed., eds. R.H. Binstock and E. Shanas, 554–85. New York: Van Nostrand Reinhold.

Jacobs, B. 1990. Aging in Politics. In *Handbook of Aging and the Social Sciences,* 3rd ed., eds. R.H. Binstock and L.K. George, 349–61. San Diego, Calif.: Academic Press.

Jahnigen, D.W., and R.H. Binstock. 1991. Economic and Clinical Realities: Health Care for Elderly People. In *Too Old for Health Care?: Controversies in Medicine, Law, Economics and Ethics,* eds. R.H. Binstock and S.G. Post, 13–43. Baltimore, Md.: Johns Hopkins University Press.

Kalish, R.A. 1979. The New Ageism and the Failure Models: A Polemic. *The Gerontologist* 19:398–407.

Kingson, E.R., B.A. Hirshorn, and J.M. Cornman. 1986. *Ties That Bind: The Interdependence of Generations.* Washington: Seven Locks Press.

Kleiman, D. 1985. Death and the Court. *New York Times* (January 19):9.

Koenig, R. 1986. As Liver Transplants Grow More Common, Ethical Issues Multiply: By Operating on the Elderly, Thomas Starzl Steps Up Patient Selection Debate. *Wall Street Journal* (October 14):1.

Kutza, E.A. 1981. *The Benefits of Old Age.* Chicago: University of Chicago Press.

La Puma, J., M. Silverstein, C. Stocking, D. Roland, and M. Siegler. 1988. Life-Sustaining Treatment: A Prospective Study of Patients with DNR Orders in a Teaching Hospital. *Archives of Internal Medicine* 148:2193–98.

——. 1989a. Columbus and Copernicus: New Wine in Old Wineskins. *Mount Sinai Journal of Medicine* 56(1):1–10.

——. 1989b. Saving a Few, Sacrificing Many—At Great Cost. *New York Times* (August 8):23.

Light, P. 1985. *Artful Work: The Politics of Social Security Reform.* New York: Random House.

——. 1989. Elderly, Affluent—and Selfish. *New York Times* (October 10):27.

Lubitz, J., and R. Prihoda. 1984. The Use and Costs of Medicare Services in the Last Two Years of Life. *Health Care Financing Review* 5(3):117–31.

Marmor, T.R. 1970. *The Politics of Medicare.* London: Routledge and Kegan Paul.

Miles, S., and Ryder, M. 1985. Limited-Treatment Policies in Long-Term Care Facilities. *Journal of the American Geriatric Society* 33:707.

Neugarten, B.L., and D.A. Neugarten. 1986. Age in the Aging Society. *Daedalus* 115(1):31–49.

New York Times/CBS News Poll. 1980. How Different Groups Voted for President. *The New York Times* (November 9):28.

——. 1982. Party Choices of Voters, 1982 vs. 1978. *New York Times* (November 8):B11.

——. 1984. Portrait of the Electorate. *New York Times* (November 8):A19.

——. 1986. Portrait of the Electorate: The Vote for House of Representatives. *New York Times* (November 6):15Y.

——. 1988. Portrait of the Electorate. *New York Times* (November 10):18Y.

Peterson, P. 1987. The Morning After. *The Atlantic* 260(4):43–69.

Post, S.G. 1991. Justice and the Elderly: Judeo-Christian Perspectives. In *Too Old For Health Care?: Controversies in Medicine, Law, Economics, and Ethics,* eds. R.H. Binstock and S.G. Post, 120–37. Baltimore, Md.: Johns Hopkins University Press.

Pratt, H.J. 1976. *The Gray Lobby.* Chicago: University of Chicago Press.

Preston, S.H. 1984. Children and the Elderly in the U.S. *Scientific American* 251(6):44–49.

Roos, N.P., P. Montgomery, and L.L. Roos. 1987. Health Care Utilization in the Years Prior to Death. *Milbank Memorial Fund Quarterly/Health and Society* 65:231–54.

Samuelson, R.J. 1978. Aging America: Who Will Shoulder the Growing Burden? *National Journal* 10:1712–17.

Schneider, E.L., and J.M. Guralnik. 1990. The Aging of America: Impact on Health Care Costs. *Journal of the American Medical Association* 263:2335–46.

Schulte J. 1983. Terminal Patients Deplete Medicare, Greenspan Says. *Dallas Morning News* (April 26):1.

Schwartz, D., and P. Reilly. 1986. The Choice Not to be Resuscitated. *Journal of the American Geriatric Society* 34:807–11.

Scitovsky, A. A. 1984. "The High Cost of Dying": What Do the Data Show? *Milbank Memorial Fund Quarterly/Health and Society* 62:591–608.

——. 1988. Medical Care in the Last Twelve Months of Life: The Relation between Age, Functional Status, and Medical Care Expenditures. *Milbank Memorial Fund Quarterly/Health and Society* 66:640–60.

Simon, H.A. 1985. Human Nature in Politics: The Dialogue of Psychology with Political Science. *American Political Science Review* 79:293–304.

Slater, W. 1984. Latest Lamm Remark Angers the Elderly. *Arizona Daily Star* (March 29):1.

Smeeding, T.M. 1990. Economic Status of the Elderly. In *Handbook of Aging and the Social Sciences*, 3rd ed., eds. R.H. Binstock and L.K. George, 362–81. San Diego, Calif.: Academic Press.

Smeeding, T.M., M.P. Battin, L.P. Francis, and B.M. Landesman, eds. 1987. *Should Medical Care Be Rationed by Age?* Totowa, N.J.: Rowman and Littlefield.

Starr, P. 1983. *The Social Transformation of American Medicine.* New York: Basic Books.

Thurow, L.C. 1985. Medicine versus Economics. *New England Journal of Medicine* 313:611–14.

Torrey, B.B. 1982. Guns vs. Canes: The Fiscal Implications of an Aging Population. *American Economics Association Papers and Proceedings* 72:309–13.

U.S. Congress. Office of Technology Assessment. 1987. *Life-Sustaining Technologies and the Elderly.* Washington.

U.S. House of Representatives. Select Committee on Aging. 1989. *Health Care Costs for America's Elderly, 1977–88.* Washington.

——. 1988. *Developments in Aging: 1987—Volume 1.* Washington.

Veatch, R. 1988. Justice and the Economics of Terminal Illness. *Hastings Center Report* 18(4):34–40.

Wisensale, S.M. 1988. Generational Equity and Intergenerational Policies. *The Gerontologist* 28:773–78.

Youngner, S., W. Lewandowski, D. McClish, B. Juknialis, C. Coulton, and E. Bartlett. 1985. Do Not Resuscitate Orders: Incidence and Implications in a Medical Intensive Care Unit. *Journal of the American Medical Association* 253:54–57.

Index to Authors

Aaron, Henry J., 70
Altman, Drew E., 67
Annas, George J., 150
Binstock, Robert H., 267
Bodenheimer, Thomas, 73, 199
Brennan, Troyen A., 246
Brook, Robert H., 230
Brown, Lawrence D., 76
Callahan, Daniel, 260
Cox, Jafna L., 158
Fuchs, Victor R., 240
Grumbach, Kevin, 199

Klein, Rudolf, 167
Kuttner, Robert, 107
Levitt, Larry, 67
Madison, Donald L., 31
Mariner, Wendy K., 128
McGlynn, Elizabeth A., 230
Oberlander, Jonathan, 5
Parrish, Geov, 119
Redmayne, Sharon, 167
Reinhardt, Uwe E., 25, 179
Sparer, Michael S., 76
Stone, Deborah, 95

About the Editors

Larry R. Churchill, PhD, holds the Ann Geddes Stahlman Chair in Medical Ethics, Department of Medicine, Center for Clinical and Research Ethics, Vanderbilt University. He also holds appointments in Vanderbilt's Divinity School and in the Department of Philosophy. From 1988 to 1998 he was chair of the Department of Social Medicine, University of North Carolina at Chapel Hill School of Medicine. His recent research is focused on justice and U.S. health policy, the ethics of research with human subjects, and the relationship between bioethics and ordinary moral experience.

Sue E. Estroff, PhD, is a professor in the Department of Social Medicine and an adjunct professor in the Departments of Anthropology and Psychiatry, School of Medicine and College of Arts and Sciences, University of North Carolina at Chapel Hill. She is the author of numerous cultural analyses of schizophrenia and other severe persistent psychiatric disorders, focusing most recently on the topics of contested identity and conflicting representations between medical and psychiatric formulations and those of people with schizophrenia. Her other current work includes cultural analysis of consent in the context of experimental fetal surgery, exploring moral quandaries in the production of knowledge, and examining the roles of social and cultural factors in violence in the lives of people with schizophrenia.

Gail E. Henderson, PhD, is a professor in the Department of Social Medicine, School of Medicine, and Adjunct Professor in the Department of Sociology, College of Arts and Sciences, University of North Carolina at Chapel Hill. Her teaching and research interests include health and inequality, health and health care in China, and research ethics. She has extensive experience with qualitative and quantitative data collection and analysis, as well as with conceptual and empirical cross-disciplinary research and analysis. In China, she has taught social science research methods to clinical epidemiologists, and conducted research ethics training workshops for HIV / AIDS researchers. Her current research focuses on ethical issues in gene transfer clinical trials and cancer genetic epidemiology studies, and understanding how research ethics committees in China and Africa oversee international collaborative research.

Nancy M. P. King, JD, is a professor in the Department of Social Medicine, University of North Carolina at Chapel Hill School of Medicine. Her scholarly interests focus on individual and policy-level decision making in health care and research, and the relationship between bioethics and law. She teaches and advises on human subjects research ethics and healthcare ethics locally, nationally, and internationally, addressing issues ranging from literature and medicine to end-of-life court decisions to genetic databases. Her current research and most recent publications address informed consent in gene transfer research.

Jonathan Oberlander, PhD, is an associate professor in the Department of Social Medicine at the University of North Carolina at Chapel Hill, where he teaches health policy in the School of Medicine and Department of Political Science. He is a Greenwall Foundation Faculty Scholar in Bioethics and the author of *The Political Life of Medicare* (University of Chicago Press). His research and teaching interests include health politics and policy, Medicare, health care reform, and medical care rationing. Current research focuses on market-based strategies for Medicare reform, the politics of incremental and state-led health reform, and a study of the Oregon Health Plan.

Ronald P. Strauss, DMD, PhD, is a professor in the Department of Social Medicine, School of Medicine, and Dental Friends Distinguished Professor and Chair, Department of Dental Ecology, School of Dentistry, University of North Carolina at Chapel Hill. He is both a sociologist of medicine and a dentist, with a research focus on stigmatization and the social impacts of chronic health problems including craniofacial anomalies and HIV/AIDS. He is the director of the Social and Behavioral Sciences Research Core of the UNC Center for AIDS Research. Current research includes an oral health disparities research project in Hawaii, a study of health promotion in low-income workplaces in eastern North Carolina, a study that examines stigma experience related to TB and HIV in south Thailand, and a multisite project that evaluates quality of life in adolescents with facial differences.

Library of Congress Cataloging-in-Publication Data
The social medicine reader.—2nd ed.
p. ; cm.
Includes bibliographical references and index.
ISBN 0-8223-3555-7 (v. 1 : cloth : alk. paper)
ISBN 0-8223-3568-9 (v. 1 : pbk. : alk. paper)
ISBN 0-8223-3580-8 (v. 2 : cloth : alk. paper)
ISBN 0-8223-3593-X (v. 2 : pbk. : alk. paper)
ISBN 0-8223-3556-5 (v. 3 : cloth : alk. paper)
ISBN 0-8223-3569-7 (v. 3 : pbk. : alk. paper)
1. Social medicine.
[DNLM: 1. Social Medicine—Collected Works.
2. Ethics, Clinical—Collected Works. 3. Health
Policy—Collected Works. 4. Professional-Patient
Relations—Collected Works. 5. Sick Role—Col-
lected Works. 6. Socioeconomic Factors—Collected
Works. 7. Terminal Care—Collected Works.
WA 31 S67803 2005] I. King, Nancy M. P.
RA418.S6424 2005   362.1'042—dc22   2005010301